WOMEN AND FATIGUE

'But, Doctor, why am I so tired?'

This was the question which Dr Marion Hilliard, a leading Canadian gynaecologist, found she was continually being asked. Her patients were so often apparently healthy women who confessed themselves ground down by life and unable to meet its challenge and its opportunities. Letters from readers of her first and highly successful book, *A Woman Doctor Looks at Love and Life* posed the same problem. In answer, therefore, she wrote this inspiring and comprehensive handbook on fatigue in women.

The fatigue problems of many types of women, adolescent girls, young mothers, career women, the middle-aged and the elderly are dealt with in turn, and for each Dr Hilliard suggests practical ways of re-organizing the limited energy available to each human being, and thus realizing quite new achievements in life. Home-making, the doctor-patient relationship, sex, nervous disorders – Dr Hilliard's scope is wide, but throughout the book she maintains her lucid style, urged on by her conviction that each and every woman can conquer fatigue. She ends on a religious note of deep conviction, entitling her final chapter 'Love God and Do as You Please'. Then, she declares, fatigue will vanish of its own accord.

WOMEN AND FATIGUE

Dr Marion Hilliard was a popular and well-loved figure in Canada. Born in Morrisburg in 1902, she graduated from the University of Toronto Medical School, where she had been a star athlete, in 1927 and did post-graduate research in Europe. For many years Chief of Obstetrics and Gynaecology at the Women's College Hospital in Toronto, she delivered over 10,000 babies, many of them called Marion after her. Before her death in 1958 she did valuable work in cancer research.

WOMEN AND FATIGUE

A Woman Doctor's Answer

DR MARION HILLIARD

PAN BOOKS LTD · LONDON

First published in Great Britain 1960 by Macmillan & Co. Ltd.

This edition published 1963 by Pan Books Ltd.
33 Tothill Street, London S.W.1.

ISBN 0 330 02279 2

2nd Printing 1969
3rd Printing 1972

Printed in Great Britain by
Cox & Wyman Ltd., London, Reading and Fakenham

CONTENTS

ACKNOWLEDGEMENTS

FOREWORD

1	'But, Doctor, Why Am I So Tired?'	11
2	It's Not All in Your Mind	16
3	Fatigue Is a Fact	27
4	Fatigue Has Many Faces	36
5	Alas, 'Tis Our Frailty	48
6	A Time to be Born and a Time to Die	67
7	Common Sense and Calories	85
8	Secrets of Happy Family Life	91
9	Too Tired to Love	104
10	Shadows Cast by Our Modern Way of Life	115
11	The Fallacy of the Short Cut to Vitality	134
12	Trapped by Her Own Adaptability	148
13	'Love God and Do as You Please'	156

INDEX

ACKNOWLEDGEMENTS

Grateful acknowledgement is made to the many friends and associates of Dr Hilliard who co-operated to make available the materials for this book and to the following individuals and organizations for permission to use ideas from broadcasts and published articles and papers: American Medical Women's Association; Maclean-Hunter Publishing Co. (*Chatelaine* Magazine); Martha Deane and Station WOR, New York; Young Women's Christian Association of Canada. Special thanks are due Miss Jennifer Dench, who typed all drafts of the manuscript.

The selection from John Masefield's *Good Friday* (*Selected Poems of John Masefield*) is used with permission of the Macmillan Company of New York, the Society of Authors of London, and Dr John Masefield, O.M.

FOREWORD

MARION HILLIARD believed fatigue to be the greatest enemy a woman ever faces. In her daily practice as Chief of Obstetrics and Gynaecology, at Women's College Hospital in Toronto, as well as in discussion following a lecture or during an interview, she found the question most often asked was 'Why am I so tired?' Letters from readers of her first book, *A Woman Doctor Looks at Love and Life*, frequently posed the same problem.

Dr Hilliard felt that helping women to overcome this devastating fatigue was 'the most challenging and rewarding part of my practice'. Her ideas sprang not only from her convictions as a medical practitioner but also from a deeply rooted personal philosophy of positive attitudes, values, and faith. It was her idea to write her second book on this topic, and she was devoting herself eagerly and enthusiastically to the project until a very few days before her death on July 15, 1958, of a rare type of cancer.

In addition to the notes and outline Marion Hilliard had made for the book, there were many other sources of material in her files – speeches, medical papers, taped radio interviews, magazine pieces, and of course case histories of actual patients.

The task of collating the material, putting it together in a cohesive and meaningful order, and bridging the gaps has been accomplished by Miss Marion O. Robinson, in collaboration with Miss Opal Boynton, both long-time friends of the author. The author's brother, Dr Irwin M. Hilliard, F.R.C.P. (C), Professor of Medicine, University of Saskatchewan, Canada, acted as consultant on the physiological aspect of fatigue and has checked the entire manuscript for medical accuracy, as Marion Hilliard had originally asked him to do.

This book in its final form then may fairly be presented as 'by Marion Hilliard'. All of the thoughts and ideas are hers, and, to a great extent, the words and the characteristic phrases and expressions.

1

'But, Doctor, Why Am I So Tired?'

IT'S VERY important for women to think, and to speak about what they are thinking. As a woman and a women's doctor for thirty years, I think a lot about women – their physical and emotional assets and liabilities, the particular joys, sorrows, blessings, and hazards life has to offer them, the particular gifts they have to offer life.

I always like the feeling of having a cause. My cause is what this book is about: helping women to understand what I have come to believe is their greatest enemy, fatigue, and helping them learn how to cope with it. I want to answer that endlessly repeated, dreary query, 'But, Doctor, why am I so tired?'

It makes me unhappy to see a woman beaten down by plain ordinary fatigue that has gone on too long. I'd rather help her become a healthy, happy woman than save a life by an operation. Any day. A woman who is chronically without energy plays hostess to an endless parade of backaches, headaches, infections. She may behave like a shrew, alienate her husband, lose her best friends. Worst of all she is without joy, with no dreams of tomorrow.

The greatest pleasure I have is seeing a woman get on

her feet physically because she has worked out an intelligent attack on her fatigue problem. She has a spring in her step and feels a sense of well-being and a little joy of living, for a change. Her whole family benefits by it. So do her friends, neighbours, and her community.

If we had enough of these blessed, enlightened females, women could really begin to learn their way around this world we have made for ourselves.

A woman's biological nature, quaintly referred to as 'frailty' in earlier centuries, makes her, to some degree, vulnerable to fatigue. Almost any woman will find times in the monthly menstrual cycle when physical and emotional reserve strength will ebb lower than usual. In the three periods of great bodily change – onset of cyclic life in adolescence, pregnancy, and the menopause – fatigue is inevitable.

Women today are tired for additional reasons. For one thing, they are struggling with their role as females; they are tired because of strenuous efforts to perform multiple services at home, on the job, and in the community.

What is a woman's role in life? Wife, mother, and home-maker? Assistant bread-winner? Career woman? Worker for community good? A combination? She can't decide. Meantime the intermingling of roles produces enormous fatigue. To top it off, she misses out on a sense of achievement because she isn't able to concentrate fully on any one of her goals.

Social changes have made a terrific impact on the home and family. Girls and boys are getting married in their late teens, often before they have had a chance to adjust fully to the biological changes of adolescence. Several million women with pre-school children are working outside their homes. More families are on the move; some even live on wheels. It is becoming more and more difficult to make a home – a place of rest, refreshment, nurture, contentment.

It is a strange paradox that in a world filled with time- and labour-saving devices we are nearly all sufferers from fatigue. The kind of fatigue I mean is a tiredness that goes on until it parlays itself into a state of apathy. Sometimes it comes from too much hard work for too many hours. Probably the mother of a family of small children is the most likely of all women in today's society to suffer from this. The wife who tries to manage a home and also go out to work is a close runner-up.

But a good deal of the fatigue comes from such unsuspected sources as loneliness, frustration, the compulsive drive of modern life. These fatigue factors are harder to deal with than the natural fatigue which results from overwork and is remedied by rest. Sometimes, in fact, they are insidiously difficult to track down.

Women can be helped by their own doctors to find out what their limits are and what causes stress in their lives. The main difficulty I have had with my patients is to get across to them that, being females and living in today's world, they must keep assessing what's going on with them and their lives. Periodic assessments can keep a man on the track with his roles as employee, husband, and father. He follows a straight line, going forward usually on the same kind of job. Then he comes home to his family. Women's lives are never like that. A woman has to shift emphases constantly among her various roles. Sometimes she has to be mostly wife, sometimes all mother, sometimes part of the community. The problem is to get sorted out; after that it's easy. Without the sorting out, the assessment, women get tired and fall by the wayside.

Sometimes after I have examined a patient and told her, 'Now, get dressed and come and talk with me,' I can just hear her, while she's getting dressed and fixing her hair, saying to herself, 'There's nothing wrong with me. I'm just taking a lot of the doctor's time. All I needed to do was pull myself together. This is a very stupid thing.' She comes back and sits down, but even before she gets settled she's opening her purse to get her car keys out. Then the following dialogue takes place:

Me: 'Now, here are your instructions. This is what you are to do.'

Patient: 'But, Doctor, there's nothing wrong with me.'

Me: 'Now, listen to what I say.'

She has a bad case of 'It's all in my mind', and I know I'm going to have to take all distractions away from her and get her to sit quietly and listen until finally she lights up and I know she's caught on.

There has to be a channel of communication between us. If either of us is too busy, the channel is blocked.

Nothing obscures and distorts the spirit as much as busyness about small things.

She may be sitting on the edge of her chair because she's preoccupied about getting home to get dinner for the family. I may be sitting on the edge of my chair because I have a patient in labour, or must go to make a speech, or get home to water the garden. We both have to get past those things. Patients don't realize that sometimes they encourage their doctors to have a take-it-or-leave-it attitude because they themselves don't take their treatment seriously.

I want you, like my patient, to catch on to the fact that if you will, you can vanquish your fatigue problem. Because this has happened so many times in my years of practice, I am practically an evangelist on the subject of fatigue, what causes women to be that way, how they can avert it, how they can treat it with good sense.

This I believe: that women of any age can not only accept, survive, and withstand, but that they can have zest for living throughout their entire lives.

2

It's Not All in Your Mind

PHYSICIANS since the time of Hippocrates have been amazed at the power of nature to heal itself, the ability of a living creature to survive, to adapt itself to its environment. On the other hand they have also been bewildered by inexplicable defeat of the total organism that is the human body, and the appearance of local disturbance without an adequate known cause.

We have had clinical evidence of a living energy that fights – and of an appalling lassitude that cannot be aroused.

I go into the recovery room at noon. The patient who was operated on at eight o'clock is still sound asleep, flat out. But the one who at ten o'clock had the most difficult operation of the day sits up and says, 'Well, Doctor, how are things?' I walk down the corridor wondering just what the difference is between my two patients. No obvious facts explain it.

Or here are two women having their babies on the same day. They are the same age, both in good health. One sails through the whole thing, reviving as she goes along. You can see the power of nature at work in her. For the other, that power wanes into exhaustion. It takes days for her to reach the point of revival that the first one got to before she left the delivery room. Again I am left asking, 'Why?'

Doctors observe many things in the course of practice that they don't know the 'why' about. Sometimes a lot of little 'whys' will add up to a big one. The most baffling and intriguing 'why' for me is this: Why doesn't the law of cause and effect operate in the same way for different people?

Childbirth or a major operation make an all-out call on a woman's total resources. Some women breeze through it. Others don't stand it well. Not because they have a low pain tolerance, but there's just something about the constitution that can't stand the assault. ('Assault' or 'insult' are technical terms we use to describe a great demand made upon the total organism.)

A few hours after a major operation one patient may sit up and ask for her lunch. Another will be in a fog for a week and require a much longer period of convalescence. It's almost as though a woman stopped producing a certain kind of energy after the operation. Another woman seems to have energy more easily available. She's the one who gets a good rest in the hospital.

The ordinary peltings of daily living affect women differently also. Two fundamentally well women may be running their homes and carrying responsible jobs. One zooms through her days exuberantly. The other accomplishes what she has to, but begins to sag in mid-afternoon. A mother of three pre-schoolers compares herself with her neighbour: 'By eight o'clock when the kids are in bed and the dinner dishes are done, I'm falling apart. But not Mary! Putting *her* children to bed is just the beginning of a big evening to her. She can stitch up a whole new outfit before midnight!'

Often these perfectly well women just aren't functioning properly. They complain of low right side backaches, headaches, profuse periods. They show up with repeated infections that you can't explain, except to say, lamely, that your patient is 'infection-prone'.

To get at the 'why' of these puzzling differences – or as much of it as we know about – we start with a little physiology review. Just hold on to your hats. Here we go.

The universal pattern of all human growth is also seen in the life of each individual person. Birth, childhood, puberty, adolescence, maturity, climacteric, old age, and death form the normal cycle for all of us.

But in each person, as in nature, there are many variations which overlay or modify the basic pattern. In any one person's reaction to a situation we may glimpse a combination of the current phase of development (adolescence, the menopause, or whatever), heredity (physical and mental attributes), and the external circumstances within which she lives.

An inherent law of development governs all phases of development in a person. Each phase is potentially present right from the beginning in the fertilized egg.

It seems incredible that every human being is, to start with, one small microscopic cell. In that cell are all his inherited characteristics, all the properties of himself.

The great powers of life are there too – the powers of reproduction and of preservation of life.

The cell divides. The various properties are divided into systems. One system develops, then another and another. At first each system goes its own way. Then a regulator – the nervous system – steps into the picture, and is given power over the others. Finally the group of glands of internal secretion develop – the pituitary, thyroid, adrenal, and sex glands. Their job is to pour substances called hormones into the blood stream.

Hormones from some glands of internal secretion affect other glands, almost as if the latter were on an assembly line. At the same time they affect and are affected by the nervous system. The upshot is that a human being is a glandular system regulated by a nervous system or, to put it another way, he is a neuroglandular system. The functioning of that system is his metabolic pattern.

Metabolism is a word we're going to use a lot, so let's get it down pat. The metabolism of a person is the biochemical changes – vital processes – which go on in living cells throughout the body. It is regulated by the neuroglandular system, controlled by the interrelationship of the nervous system and the endocrine system. Metabolism produces energy.

The working relationship of the nervous and endocrine system, which determines your metabolic pattern, is so close the two just cannot be separated. Usually the nervous system has the upper hand, so to speak, and is in control of the endocrine system, but in those periods of life when glandular changes are taking place, such as adolescence and menopause, glandular activities are temporarily not quite under the control of the nervous system. This can make people speak or cry louder than they normally do, and may, for the moment, affect their judgement about getting into arguments about non-essentials! Normally, however, the nervous system acts as the great correlator of body processes.

This nervous system, by the way, is not just a cloverleaf of sensory fibres and motor responses. It is not passive. It is an intelligent, thinking, feeling, emotionally active cell structure. It is sensitive to inner changes, sensitive to the environment and to the various stresses in that environment.

Your metabolic pattern functions on its own. Certain things it will do in your life are predictable, for they are inherent back in that single cell with which you started life. It is inherent in the female cell, for instance, that the change we call menopause will occur in middle age. We don't know why it occurs, we just know it's inevitable. That's why I say hormones act on their own. It's as though they sat up and said to themselves, 'Now we will have adolescence,' or, 'Now it's time for the menopause.'

The timing and intensity of daily changes in neuroglandular activity are different in different people. You might say that each person has his own system of gears and shifts. This accounts for the observable differences of metabolic patterns.

Some people wake up at six o'clock in the morning,

merry as a coot and ready for anything. At ten o'clock at night they are bushed. That's one kind of metabolic pattern. Another person can't really start the day till she's had two cups of coffee and has wandered around long enough to get everything in focus. At 10 p.m. she's just hitting her stride. That's another kind of metabolic pattern.

One of the glands you're born with is the pituitary. This gland starts up much of the endocrine production by stimulating other glands of internal secretion. It is thought to have a daily rhythm and to be more active at an earlier hour of the day in some people than in others. This may explain why your neighbour is a ball of fire at 7 a.m. while you have your maximum energy at 9 p.m.

You were born with it, this metabolic pattern. The very complex single cell that is you at the beginning holds all the characteristics you have inherited from your family and your family's family. Along with other things, like the colour of your eyes or hair, you inherit your hormone system, your nervous system, *and* the way they interact.

This is really the beginning answer to the questions that come up so often:

'Why don't I have the energy my neighbour (or mother – or sister) has?'

'Why can't I seem to manage this type of work?'

'Why am I too tired to go any place in the evening?'

And someone else says, 'I was born tired.' So, maybe she was. She was born with a different type of metabolic pattern. It is a fact that we all have different rhythms of energy production.

But we – you – can do something about it.

Take a couple of people I know. Frances is one of those quick people. She reacts quickly, understands quickly. She lights up like a candle over a new idea, even though her enthusiasm may not hold for long. Edith lights up more slowly. It takes her a while to become aware of what's going on. Then she builds up more and more enthusiasm until she's ready to go. By that time Frances has gone on to something else.

I suppose you might say that people like Frances are superficial, have no mind, don't really think. Not necessarily. Each nervous system has its own pattern and rhythm. You and I must learn what our pattern is.

The quality of activity in your body varies even under ordinary circumstances, such as when the day really begins for you and when it comes to an end. But at certain important periods of a woman's life the activity of the nervous and glandular systems undergoes a great change, often producing somewhat erratic types of behaviour.

At these special periods of life we know now we can expect outward and visible signs of tremendous physiological change. This is why study of adolescence, the prenatal period and menopause have taught us much about hormone activity. For example, the observation that arthritis lessens, sometimes disappears, during pregnancy led to the treatment of arthritis by cortisone. (I have to remind myself now that there really was a time when we still did not know the effect of cortisone in the treatment of arthritis.)

By now it must be apparent that in a marriage of two metabolic patterns that don't gee there is bound to be a certain amount of emotional disturbance. To understand it, you first have to realize that the behaviour does not spring from wilfulness or shallowness – it's the way the person is made. Whether you call it a metabolic rhythm or a psychological phenomenon this is a fact that holds true. When your husband says, 'I can't help it. That's the way I'm made,' he just might be right.

Take the low-metabolism wife and the energetic husband. One such patient of mine, with the added disadvantage of a compulsion to keep a perfect house, was married to a gay blade who loved to go dancing. Finally backache, flooding at menstruation, and a parade of infections put her at the end of her rope – and into my office.

'You'll have to face up to making a choice,' I told her. 'My vote is that you let some of the household chores go, so you can have fun with your husband.'

Her face was a picture of horror and I knew she was mentally shuddering at the prospect of a long conveyer belt of rough-dry clothing, undone dishes, and dusty coffee tables. But she gamely agreed to try. I didn't see her for almost a year after that.

'I can see I don't have to ask you if you're well and happy,' I said, after one look at her. 'Tell me, what did you do about your housekeeping schedule?'

'Well, the house is something less than a showpiece,

I must say,' she replied placidly. 'But the people in it are all in fine shape, including me. I feel better now that I'm being me instead of trying to be three other people.'

A high-metabolism wife has her troubles, too. The bride of a man fifteen years her senior felt her marriage was heading for disaster. An early riser, she was at her best in the morning – cheerful, alert, and talkative. Her husband, a charming conversationalist and something of a wit, rose reluctantly, came to breakfast gloomily, and sat silent and unresponsive. But at night no party could last long enough for him; she herself could have folded early and never gone to the party at all. She had begun to brood. Could she make him happy after all? Maybe her friends who had warned against marrying 'an older man' had been right.

When I suggested that their disparate metabolic cycles could account for their differences, this intelligent young woman latched on to the information eagerly. Now instead of lamenting the fact that he can't seem to face a new day with her, she turns on his hot shower and leaves an eye-opener cup of coffee within reach. Both help raise the body temperature as a starter on the day. Wisely, too, she has learned to save time for a late afternoon nap on party nights, to keep her own metabolic pattern in the groove with her husband's.

With some people, the mind is willing but the metabolism is weak. The mind has more drive than the metabolic state can support. This person plans more than she can possibly do in the time she allows. She must learn to

24

be more realistic. Not that she should give up her dreams and plans – far from it! But she can space them out over longer periods and plan the energy-demanding things for the times she has learned she has the most energy available. This saves frustration, which in itself is very fatigue-producing!

The true relation between energy demand and energy production within ourselves is not yet well understood in the medical world. Energy may have its own habit pattern, may even *be* a habit pattern. We all know that the busiest people are the ones most likely to take on new projects and responsibilities. If such an active person were to key her life to a lower pitch, she might find she had less energy instead of more. As one colleague of mine puts it, 'It may well be that running upstairs creates energy as well as using it.' For the present we must come back to the fact that each of us has a limit with which we must become well acquainted.

In spite of our meagre knowledge in some areas, doctors observe in the lives of their patients truths of human experience which might be called facts of life. And many people discover these truths for themselves. One is that though fatigue patterns differ, each has its basis in the constitution and metabolic functioning of the person.

Further than that, the same people have different patterns at different times. The same mother may handle a family row between the same children at two different times, feeling no fatigue at one time and complete exhaustion at the other. The first time it was 8 a.m., when she was feeling fresh, the second at 8 p.m., when she was finishing the dishes after a day of house cleaning.

The key to knowledge of your store of energy is a first-rate assessment of your metabolic pattern. Look at your mother, father, aunts, uncles, and grandparents, because you inherited your pattern from them. Find out what those inheritances are.

3

Fatigue Is a Fact

For well over twenty years I collected observations from among my patients on the fatigue patterns which grow out of metabolic rhythms.

Then came the second most exciting moment of my years in the medical profession. (The first was in 1922, when I was in medical school at the University of Toronto. That was the year that insulin was discovered, at the University, by Banting and Best. Many people today owe their lives to this discovery. I will never forget the excitement. It put a whole new dimension on my experience as a medical student.)

But that's another story. My second biggest thrill was the night I heard Dr Hans Selye talk about his ideas on stress. In his search for a new female hormone, he had accidentally fallen across a new line of endeavour. His subsequent searching has cast light on things doctors have talked about since the beginning of medical history, including my wonderings about my patient with the terrific operation who could sit up two hours later in the recovery room and begin asking questions.

As Dr Selye talked, I felt at last we had the key to

unlock the secret of nature's power to revive – and also of the lassitude that defies arousal. We could begin to answer the question of why certain individuals had or did not have energy. We were getting at the principle that underlies the reaction of the patient to disease or disaster.

At this point we add another indispensable word to our vocabulary, along with 'metabolism'. The word is 'stress'.

Stress, as Dr Selye puts it, is 'the rate of wear and tear on the body'. 'Stressors' or 'stress factors' are those activities or emotions which produce the wear and tear.

We cannot live without continuously experiencing some degree of stress. It may be pleasant as well as unpleasant, so stress is not necessarily bad for us. 'Even sheer joy,' says Dr Selye, 'is enough to activate the body stress mechanism to some extent.'

The degree of stress and the length of time it's applied are the significant characteristics when one relates stress to an understanding of fatigue. Dr Selye has invented a term, the 'general adaptation syndrome', to describe the sequence in which the body reacts to activity in its environment. First there is the 'alarm', then the 'stage of resistance', and then the 'stage of exhaustion'.

What has this to do with our neuroglandular system, our producer of energy? Suppose your body is subjected to some great stress – intense cold, a burn, an operation. It reacts immediately to the 'alarm' and begins to 'adapt' to the stress. If the strain is too prolonged or

28

too intense, and your body is not able to reinforce itself through your nervous system and the effect of the hormones, the stage of resistance passes and the stage of exhaustion begins. First you adapt, then you feel fatigued, then exhausted – it's a matter of degree and timing.

Experiments conducted over short periods of time in dramatic circumstances illustrate the general adaptation syndrome. Put a person in a cold atmosphere. At first his body will adapt and he can get along. After a certain number of minutes he will reach a stage of fatigue. If he stays there longer still – a matter of hours – he will become exhausted. His glands of internal secretion will no longer function as they did when he was in a room at the temperature his body requires.

The time element is important to your doctor who is trying to treat and cure you of fatigue. When a person is exhausted, the hormonal glands cannot easily be restimulated to undertake their function. Naturally your doctor is interested in your family background, because he wants to know something about those inherited characteristics we talked about. If you have a fatigue problem, your 'stress history' is important to him, too. What's been going into your life, day by day, over a long period of time reveals the link between cause and effect.

The link is easy to see in the person who has had a sudden, severe shock. The effect, in the form of a disorganization of the endocrine system, may appear in a matter of hours. The link is more difficult to discern when the cause of exhaustion has been accumulating over a long period of time.

I remember a patient who came to me with complaints of extreme menopausal fatigue. In the course of our interview I found she was drinking too much, eating too little. A smouldering resentment against her husband, who had been stricken with a chronic illness fifteen years earlier, was very near the surface. My treatment included a mandate to arrange for a little help to lessen the burden of caring for her husband, although I was foolish enough to be puzzled about why she was so exhausted at this particular point, since the three children she had brought up almost single-handed because of her husband's illness had now grown and left home.

As she grew more rested and relaxed and I grew to know her better, I realized she had been accumulating fatigue for fifteen years, but that a combination of pride in her self-sufficiency, a good constitution, and her real devotion to her husband and children, with perhaps a little touch of martyrdom thrown in, had kept her from paying much attention to herself. Not only had she overdrawn on her store of energy, but she was continuing to expend it unnecessarily by supervising her married daughter's menu-making, food shopping, and cooking. Fatigue had made such inroads on her perspective that she resented her helpless husband and felt hurt when her daughter indicated that she would prefer to handle by herself the culinary department in her own home. Once my patient evaluated what had happened to her and what she was doing to herself and her family, she began a masterful job of re-educating herself. At the end of four months she was back on her feet, happy at the vastly improved relationships she enjoyed with her family members.

The highs and lows of stressful activities or emotions do not change your metabolic cycle, but they can speed it up or slow it down. Sometimes being in love or getting steamed up over an exciting new job can inspire the metabolic machinery to work beyond its usual capacity, temporarily raising the metabolism. An attractive young patient of mine with a typical low-energy pattern began suffering extreme fatigue in her mid-twenties, following a disappointing love affair. Life had become so distasteful to her that she was not eating enough of the right kind of food. While following a regime we had agreed on, including better diet, relaxing recreation, and rest, she met another man and became engaged. What with this new and pleasant 'stress factor' and her restorative regime, she quickly regained her normal energy and more.

Generally speaking, the human system seems to be able to manage more additional energy production for a short period, less additional for a long period.

Changing gears abruptly sometimes has a dramatic effect on metabolism. A person who has been living under great pressure which is suddenly and completely relieved feels a let-down, and may even be temporarily exhausted. I have seen women who have cared for a family member during a long illness react this way after the patient has died or recovered enough to go away for convalescence. We all have such experiences in lesser degree when we have completed a long piece of work, stage-managed a big wedding, or finished examinations after a long, gruelling course of study.

Fatigue is something you can enjoy and not be afraid of. The normal fatigue that follows accomplishment – regardless of whether the process has been pleasant or unpleasant – *should* be enjoyed. Rest, relax, and you will be revived by one good night's sleep.

It's the fatigue you have accumulated, the fatigue that's too great to be dispersed by normal rest or a night or two of good sleep, that can spell trouble for you.

This kind of fatigue can happen to the woman who has filled her social or business schedule too full, just as it can to the woman who is nursing an invalid or caring for a family of small children. Not only fretting and worrying but sometimes joy can lead to a state of exhaustion. The woman who 'does too much', even though she loves every minute of it, is wearing out her adrenal glands. Maybe not as fast as she would with too many unpleasant chores, but she is still heading for fatigue.

Among my favoured prescriptions for preventing fatigue is this: learn to change pace. Whether you are a young housewife with a constant, dreary, never-ending round of chores, or a working woman who keeps house too, or a middle-aged or older woman whose years of steamed-up driving to make a home and bring up children are past, find a way to change pace. Some need to slow down; others need to speed up. A quiet half-hour a day with a book, a shift to your hobby at the end of the working day, a job, volunteer or paid, that takes you into the hurly-burly of life a few hours a week – any of these may help. The important thing is to get in the groove with it, get a congenial rhythm. Each person has to find her own ways.

'What trouble do you have with women?' a radio interviewer once asked me. Instinctively I salute women's intelligence, their fortitude and endurance, the strength of their love for their families, so I had to think for a minute. Then I said my difficulty with my women patients is that they don't seem to understand themselves. They either do not understand or are not aware of their metabolic patterns. Though they are tremendously adaptable, they don't understand the stress factors in their environment well enough to adapt themselves happily to their time of life and their day-to-day life.

I've said that the key to knowledge of your store of energy is thoroughgoing appraisal of your metabolic pattern. Now I add that the real secret of happiness is the adjustment of that pattern to the stresses in your life.

Ask yourself these questions: When do I have energy? How long does it last? How long can it keep renourishing itself under different kinds of strain? How does my energy vary in the daily cycle and the monthly cycle?

Then take a look at your surroundings to see what the stress factors are. Assess these stresses in your life to see which forces are creating a struggle in your metabolic pattern. Remember that for most people some stress is a good thing, a stimulant creating demand for energy.

For most women, work, whether at home or on a job outside the home, is one of the big factors. Normally it is a stimulating factor to which women adapt and which leads to happiness. But when a woman gets to the point where work becomes a beating-down type of thing, her body goes from adaptation to fatigue. Analysis of the work situation will show whether there are multiple stresses causing a fatigue problem, or one or two fatigue-producing factors that must be dealt with. One of my patients who used to suffer from chronic fatigue is a professional woman who loved her job but spent half of her waking hours in a state of tension because of her boss, who was frequently, unpredictably, and often unreasonably, irritable. In a showdown with herself, she decided he probably would not change but she would put up with it as cheerfully as possible for the sake of a job she liked and did well. The decision in itself helped relax her tension. Eventually the stress she felt from working with a cranky boss diminished to manageable proportions.

Though any responsible and demanding business position is a stress factor, I am inclined to think it wouldn't be in the running compared with the job of a woman who has a three-year-old and a new set of twins. In the days when I was doing a good deal of obstetrics, up night after night, I sometimes felt I was really tired. Then I'd remember one of my patients with twins and be bright as a dollar again! But more about tired young mothers later.

So here you are with a certain kind of body structure which reacts in a certain kind of way to give you your own particular metabolism. From your environment, both pleasant and unpleasant stresses are continually coming at you. You know that you react to those stress factors first by adapting. If they are too prolonged or too intense you will become fatigued, then exhausted.

Glandular change is part of the force of life, the rhythm of living in which we are born, grow up, grow old, and die. As long as we live, we are reacting to stresses around us and within us. We must learn our own limits so that we can perform within them. This is not an excuse. It is a fact. Maybe it is a challenge. Certainly it is the beginning of wisdom.

4

Fatigue Has Many Faces

THE INFINITE variety of ways in which fatigue shows itself is astounding. It may be by some nervous symptom, such as a skin rash, or by a menstrual disorder, or by a real disturbance of the blood vessels, chest, or joints. Nearly always the symptoms are slight rather than dramatic, which makes it confusing for the doctor. No wonder I keep drumming away at my fatigue theme song: fatigue makes people unnecessarily uncomfortable and unhappy, and besides, it complicates a doctor's job.

Not every patient is aware of having gotten herself into a state of fatigue. Even the people who complain of feeling tired often have no idea how they got that way. I cherish for every woman the ability to tell when fatigue she herself could control is producing nagging little symptoms and making inroads on her happiness.

At least ten times a day I hear the 'why-am-I-so-tired?' question from a patient who is sure there is something terribly wrong with her. She doesn't start out with it; she ends up with it, after she has told me her symptoms and I have examined her. It's the tone of voice that tells me this isn't the kind of tiredness you have after a long day's work when you ease yourself into bed and it feels so good along your back. It's a kind of bleat, with overtones of yearning, depression, loneliness. The patient has no light in her eye, no carefree gaiety, hardly any ability left to feel joy or happiness.

Whether she's arrived at this state of exhaustion by way of a long period of overwork, or whether she has a nagging fatigue which keeps her shopping around for a magician of a doctor – while her husband grows more impatient daily – the first important thing is to help her get some self-respect.

She may be any age. She may be single, married, widowed, divorced. She may be caring for small children, working outside the home, living in a city apartment, a suburban split-level, or on a farm. Whatever these circumstances may be, she has a particular kind of metabolism, just as she has a particular colour of eyes and hair, and she is subject to stresses. She may live with very fatigue-producing stresses which she does not recognize as such. When we get beyond the worrisome symptoms and talk about the details of her daily life, clues pour forth. Eventually the clues begin to fit together, and she is able to look at the life she is living with a more objective eye. Finding there is something she can do about herself gives her hope and self-confidence.

Women must learn to be aware of the fact that they have special fatigues born of their female biology. This is so basic that I have given a whole chapter to discussion of it. The languid adolescent girl, the pregnant girl who can't keep her eyes open, the exhausted mother, the bone-weary woman in middle age and menopause – all are typical fatigue portraits in the minds' eye of the women's doctor.

Menstrual function is the outward and visible sign of the state of a woman's total metabolism, and fatigue is a cause, not a result, of menstrual disturbance. The most dramatic illustration of this I ever saw was in Greece following World War II. When I visited there in 1951 I was asked to examine and recommend treatment for women who were having all sorts of irregularity of menstrual function. I learned that during the war, when hunger was prevalent and the nutritional level so low that many people died of starvation, most of the women stopped menstruating; the young girls reaching puberty did not start. At the time of my examinations, girls of eighteen and nineteen were just showing signs of starting the menstrual cycle, and women were suffering from a variety of menstrual difficulties. Though they had survived the starvation years, the fatigue produced by prolonged inadequate diet and extraordinary stress had played havoc with their female functioning.

Different constitutions have different ways of showing the strain and stress of emotional life. Some young girls have headaches. Some are so nauseated in the morning that they can hardly make it to the office. Some have pain in their menstrual periods, and some have pain low down on the right side.

Recently an eighteen-year-old girl came in to my office for a premarital examination. She was accompanied by, or perhaps I should say brought in by, her mother. This extremely attractive child had 'pain down the right side', said the mother. She had decided there was something wrong with the girl's ovaries. It was obvious she was going to give me a chance to confirm her diagnosis. I also sensed immediately that this mother was like a drowning woman with the blessed relief of a shore in sight because her daughter was going to be married. It did not take long to discover that the real motive in bringing her daughter to me was to find out whether or not the girl was still a virgin.

'I'm coming to see you because my mother insisted on it,' the girl told me defiantly. I liked her attitude. At least we were going to grapple with the problem quickly. I went ahead with the usual questioning and examination. Her organs of reproduction were absolutely normal, but she was too thin and I could feel that the walls of her abdomen and all the organs were taut, pulled to a tight thin line.

The kind of pain she described is common and practically never associated with the ovaries. It may be caused by the way a person stands or sits. More often it is due to tension, I was almost certain that this girl was under extreme tension. The look in her eyes told me this was no ecstatic bride-to-be. She was apprehensive, guarded, and afraid. When I suggested that maybe she was excited about getting married, her eyes filled with tears.

'I'm sure it's going to be all right and I'll be terribly happy when the time comes,' she said. That was all.

While my patient dressed, I had a little conference with her mother. Though I told her her daughter was quite normal but showed signs of great strain which was the reason for the pain, she pressed to know if the child was 'all right'. Her meaning was quite obvious. Anger flowed through me.

'This is really not for me to tell you, since your daughter is of age. I would like to say that your attitude is one I don't care for. Yes, your daughter is not only a virgin, but a lovely girl that a mother can be proud of. I have a hunch her tremendous strain is caused by your attitude towards her marriage. Why have you been so anxious?'

'She's been going with this boy for three years,' she defended herself. 'They see each other constantly. I admit I have been worried.'

I took a deep breath. 'I think you've been worrying about the wrong thing. If your daughter has been going steady since she was fifteen and now at eighteen is going to marry the same boy, you should be concerned that she may never know what a deep, true adult love is like.'

This mother was eager for her daughter to marry because she would be relieved of responsibility for the girl's happiness in life. I was incensed that a grown woman would take the view that raising a teen-age daughter to be an adult meant only getting her to the altar with her virginity intact.

'Raising a girl to be a woman means helping her understand the responsibilities and possibilities of adulthood, and developing herself so she can cope with them,' I told her. 'Your daughter's tensions of uncertainty about her marriage are causing her pain.'

I told them both that I felt the marriage should be postponed until the daughter was less tired, had no pain, and had a little chance to grow up and try this most important relationship with a few tests. I hope my advice was followed, but I doubt it.

The woman no man understands is generally a tired woman. She's unpredictable. She changes her mind. What seems on the surface to be a small added chore or responsibility is greeted as The Last Straw.

The man who wants to learn to understand a woman should know that she is just as unpredictable to herself as to anyone else. The uneven rise and fall of available energy is a complete mystery to her until she makes a real study of herself and her energy patterns. He should know that the uncertainty reaches a peak in menopause, and should try, in imagination at least, to understand what it's like never to know exactly how you are going to feel; what you can depend on; whether your energy is going to be up, down, or completely missing; when you are going to feel unreasonably like biting someone's head off, and when you're going to be chiefly concerned with your own splitting head.

Most women have to make a choice of how they will spend their energy. A woman can be an excellent cook and housekeeper. She can have a family and do a grand job of bringing up her children. She can entertain charmingly. She can keep herself tastefully clothed and beautifully groomed. She can be a joyous and exuberant sex partner. Each of these takes energy. Inevitably she will 'major' in one or two and 'minor' in the others.

Women are constantly making these choices, whether they realize it or not. When they learn to know themselves well and make conscious choices, they make more sense to other people, including husbands.

'Doctor-shopping' is sometimes a symptom of fatigue. The woman who goes from doctor to doctor is usually searching for reassurance, not about a symptom, but what lies behind the symptom. A friend has cancer; she begins to be afraid she has it too. A radio or TV programme reminds her that she has a pain in the stomach, a headache, or a backache; she decides she must go see about it.

Of course a doctor always has to deal with the symptom first. But I have learned to sit down with a patient in the consulting room and say, 'Well, your back is all right. How are you getting along with your sister-in-law?' Sometimes it's a mother-in-law. I have to find out what's causing that backache.

Sometimes a patient feels this is impertinent. She starts on a round of other doctors in her quest for reassurance. Other patients get a glimmer of light from our conversation and figure things out for themselves, or seek the help of a minister or psychiatrist – someone who can help fill the need they feel within themselves.

Blessed is she who, when she feels the need for reassurance, can sit down with herself and say, 'Now, this is what my real difficulty is.'

Fatigue often wears the face of frustration. Over and over again I have seen this in women who are trying to achieve the impossible, or avoid the inevitable. In women who are trying too hard to accomplish the not-impossible I have seen it too, particularly in the work I have done on infertility. This is a special interest of mine. I know of no more exciting or rewarding field of investigation.

Infertility involves a very common form of frustration. Many, many women are not able to become pregnant when they and their husbands want to start their families.

It is possible for a physically perfect man and woman to be unable to produce a child. It is also possible for another physically perfect couple to defy all the rules of ovulation and rhythm. All other couples come between these two extremes.

When a man and woman marry, they can have no idea whether they will be fertile or not. If they come from large families they take it for granted they will have no difficulty, but this does not always hold true. Of course every couple should go to a doctor before marriage to see that they are both in good physical condition, then when they are ready to have a child the wife should return to make sure she is physically normal. The average length of time it takes a woman to become pregnant is six to nine months. If after a year she is still not pregnant, a thoroughgoing investigation should be made of both husband and wife.

I stress the time element because in my practice I have known tragic cases where months and even years of heart-searching and self-blame preceded the patient's seeking my help. Many of these situations were easily cured. The deep unhappiness had been entirely unnecessary. Among these, the cases that come most readily to mind are the women who can scarcely bring themselves to talk about their married lives because their marriages have never been consummated. It is generally believed that this problem occurs rarely, but I see at least one such woman every month of the year.

Whether these couples have been married six months or twelve years, they live in an atmosphere of defeat in which shame is one of the main ingredients. Naturally it is expected that marriage will be consummated on the wedding night or shortly afterwards. But as the days and months, and then years, pass, the problem becomes such an enormous disaster that neither husband nor wife can bear to mention it.

I can never understand why it is assumed in these cases that the difficulty is due to the wife's nervousness and tenseness. If these factors are present, they are results, not causes. In my experience, the cause is almost always a physical one, a particularly large fibrous hymen which makes consummation impossible. If there is no congenital abnormality, these cases are quickly and easily remedied.

Another sad case of infertility I encounter is the girl who has had an abortion or an illegitimate child. Often these women carry around with them an overwhelming load of secret guilt. They may feel their inability to have a baby in marriage is a judgement on them for what happened in their youth. This is such a pitiful and misguided attitude. God does not judge in this way, ever. It is true that guilt over an indiscretion might create enough tension in a woman to prevent her from becoming pregnant. But a careful examination of the pelvic organs can give a first practical answer to the haunting question, 'Is there anything wrong with me?'

Then there is the woman who wants a baby because the foundations of her marriage are crumbling. She feels she can cement the cracks by having a child. My advice to this type is always the same: fix the marriage up first. Having a baby may be an initial boost, but later it puts an extra load on the relationships, and the marriage is in much more danger of breaking down. If it does, the baby is the real sufferer.

Sometimes I have a patient who considers having a baby a challenge she must meet. Usually extremely self-centred, this woman feels she has not fulfilled her destiny until she does.

I believe there is a fundamental principle in dealing with the life force: if you *demand* what you want, you almost always lose. Pushing your own small immediate wishes without thought for a total plan seldom results in real happiness or fulfilment.

A woman who lives in an intimate suburb, small town, or rural area has an additional hazard in remaining childless: she lives in a goldfish bowl, and if she doesn't become pregnant when the community thinks she should, she must face the gossip of older women, the prying and chit-chat of younger ones. This adds to feelings of frustration and unfulfilment.

The woman may not at first find a doctor who has the

time, interest, and knowledge to help her discover the cause of her childlessness, but she must persevere; some place there will be one who is interested and who does know.

Fertility has a whimsical quality about it. Just when you are counting on its absence, there it is. There's an old wives' tale that women in the menopause become more fertile. This is nonsense. The truth is that these women have given up all thought of becoming pregnant (and so have their friends!) so the whole thing comes as a surprise to everyone and, of course, creates more of a stir.

However, it is also true that a woman can become more fertile at any age, once she has finally been able to conceive. I always tell this to a mother who has tried for some time before becoming pregnant, when she comes for her final postnatal examination. I advise her to wait six months or so before trying again. As she leaves my office, I know she's muttering to herself, 'What does she think I am? I'll never be stupid and wait again.'

This is the one whose friends will be puzzling over the teacups someday about why she and her husband planned the way they did. I can just hear them – 'They waited so long for the first child, then had a second one within a year!'

Yes, fatigue has many faces. The frustrated, the bored, the lonely, those who suffer from inability to love or make love. The genuinely overworked. Those who try to be all things to all people. Those who live with secret fear or guilt; those who live with uncertainty.

We must look within ourselves and find the way to the love, joy, happiness, and confidence which will release energy for our use.

5

Alas, 'Tis Our Frailty

'*Alas, our frailty is the cause, not we!*
For such as we are made of, such we be.'
TWELFTH NIGHT, ACT II, SCENE 2.

Mr SHAKESPEARE knew a thing or two about women. Sometimes I wonder if, like me, he had his tongue in his cheek when he wrote of frailty in women. Maybe, like me, he was impressed with something else about them – their fortitude.

I have thousands of memories associated with women's fortitude. Once, during the war, I delivered a very young woman. It was her first baby. Her husband was in the Merchant Marines and we had no idea where he was. She displayed such courage in a difficult delivery that I have never forgotten her. And I have never forgotten her mother, who stayed right with her. We were all in this thing together. I remember feeling deeply how a woman in female difficulties can draw a special kind of strength from other women.

I know a girl – not an extraordinary person at all – who gets up every morning at half past five to get her husband's breakfast. She's quite sure that her husband will drive his bus more safely if she does this faithfully. Small acts of courage are important, too.

Then I think of a young nurse who pinned me down one day when we were making rounds. 'Doctor, when are you going to tell them that she has cancer?' she said, her eyes deep with pity and concern. I was ashamed. I had been putting off the hard task of telling the husband and the father of a twenty-two-year-old woman that she could not possibly get well.

Maybe woman's fortitude is born of her frailty. Certainly her very femaleness endows her with power, even as it imposes limitations upon her.

A woman is a female all her life. From the time she is born until she dies, wherever she goes, whatever she does, her essential being and behaviour will be determined by her female nature. From little girlhood she enters the years of erratic growth and development which we call adolescence. Then she matures into a child-bearing person. For some women, this is a time when the power of desire emerges and finds the beauty of fulfilment. For others, it is a period of lesser acceptance and resignation. This chapter draws to a close and she enters another period of uncertainty, a time of apparently never-ending variation in nervous stamina and emotional control – the menopause. Then come the productive years of energy and true fulfilment of life for all women.

This is quite a variety programme. It calls for women to play many roles in a lifetime. First, the flirt. I hope the current rage for going steady has not permanently out-dated this role. In my day, playing the field was a most amazing, exciting game!

Then the role unfolds into the part of the sweetheart – the wife – the mother. After that, a happy woman retains the best of each role. Wisdom and experience give her the strength to woo, to yield, to give, to receive – and to remain mistress of herself.

Fatigue is not peculiar to women, but women have particular fatigues, born of their own biology. Sex glands are a part of the neuroglandular system whose functioning produces energy in a human being. In a woman, glandular changes attendant upon the monthly menstrual cycle and the female life cycle result in differences in metabolism, and thus in varying amounts of available energy.

Whatever her personal life story turns out to be, a woman's body prepares itself for childbearing. For some thirty years she lives a cyclic kind of life. Then she must give it up and gradually establish a different kind of physical vigour. These are female facts of life.

Three times in her life – in adolescence, at pregnancy and at the menopause – a woman's metabolism is in a state of erratic excitement. These are the times when her store of energy rises and falls capriciously, the times when fatigue, if not handled with understanding, humour and intelligence, can become a serious problem.

The first time a woman encounters the particular kind of fatigue that comes from endocrine changes is when she is an adolescent. Between the ages of eleven or twelve, as she enters her cyclic life of menstruation and fertility, until about the age of seventeen, when her glandular state has stabilized again, her glands change and her entire nervous system goes through a time of up-heaval. This, along with spurts of physical growth, pro-duces her heavy-eyed attitude about getting up in the morning, and often a malaise towards the chores which she regards as the least attractive.

Not only do teen-agers sleep heavily through the alarm and repeated summonses from other family mem-bers (though possibly not the faint sound of the tele-phone ringing several rooms away!), but because of glandular changes they also have emotional highs and lows, sometimes take a distorted view of life, are often over-sensitive to criticism or what they believe to be interference from the adult world. It is a blessing that at all ages, including this one, Nature's changes manifest themselves in comical ways. It makes it easier for every-one to live through it!

When I think of teen-agers I have known, I remember the great problem of how to fit everything in: studying for Latin examination, practising cheer-leading for Saturday's big game, getting together with a school-mate to compare notes on what to wear to the party, making an urgent phone call to smooth out a misunder-standing, washing the dinner dishes, getting mother to help fix the hem of the skirt that's absolutely the thing to wear to school tomorrow. Somehow all of it always has to be done in a short period of time!

To the teen-ager the world is a wonderful, exciting

place, full of new things to learn, people to meet, places to go. This is real.

This wondrous time of life is also a good time to learn about the laws of stress. Just so much excitement and just so many new experiences can be absorbed in a given length of time. Then a person runs low on the ability to react, and shortly becomes too fatigued to take in anything. In this period of rapid growth and change which affect the entire physical body and personality, a wise young person begins to learn about his or her own energy quota and plan activities accordingly.

This is where parents can help. In my own small sphere of influence I carry on a constant propaganda campaign to the effect that mothers and fathers, though they feel impelled to follow the modern vogue for parental permissiveness in some matters, must take responsibility for helping boys and girls learn the important things about successful living. A sensible rule or two can be an aid to learning.

For one thing, a teen-age girl needs an 'early to bed' rule for school nights. It is necessary to protect her health. When I say bedtime, I mean that pin curls are up, radio off, and she is in bed ready to go to sleep. From a health point of view, I'm much more concerned about the way girls diddle their time away on nights when they can go to bed than about the late hours they keep by going to the movies, dating or baby-sitting.

Learning to be a woman is an exciting and absorbing course of study. Whether she knows it or not, a teen-age girl is taking a first step towards happy womanhood by obeying her body's demands for extra rest in this first period of female change. It will be easier when she comes to the second period, pregnancy, because she will have learned the beginning lesson of living harmoniously with her female nature.

A woman is different when she's pregnant. Maybe she feels better, maybe worse, but she's bound to feel different.

Some ride through pregnancy on a cloud of euphoria. They love life; they have energy beyond their usual quota; they may be warm for the first time in their lives; they hardly feel fatigue. These are the ones about whom people say, 'Motherhood becomes her, so she will probably be a wonderful mother.'

Alas, it 'ain't necessarily so'. The change in her has to do with differences in hormone balance and metabolism which accompany pregnancy. After the baby is born, she will return to exactly the state she was in before; her normal metabolism will reassert itself.

Other women are really quite droopy and dreary. They have a biased outlook on life; they have no energy; they are chilly most of the time and don't enjoy their food. Far from feeling like moving mountains, they can hardly move from chair to chair. These are the ones who secretly or openly vow, 'never again'. And sometimes their husbands do too.

But this type can find comfort and cheer in the fact that she, too, will return to her normal metabolism, once the baby comes.

It is too bad that what happens to the metabolism in

pregnancy is so unpredictable, but it is. That's the reason I nearly always advise a girl not to become pregnant until she has been married for at least a few months. It is no help to a marriage which hasn't quite got under way yet for a husband to try to cope with the fact that his bride is really not interested in getting dinner, really not interested in getting up in the morning. And, in fact, is just not interested.

It's wise, too, for a husband and wife to have time to learn their own particular technique of lovemaking. Then, if there's a temporary lapse when the wife is pregnant, they can have a happy memory of what it was like, and a warm knowledge that it will be that way again.

A pregnant woman in this day and age knows she is going through a wonderful, normal process. And she knows it will end. Not many profound life experiences have such definite time limits set on them! No matter what the beginning of a pregnancy was like, under what shadow it started, I have never known a pregnant woman who wasn't eagerly awaiting her child. Even those who are saying, 'never again'. Because there is always anticipation and joy in the expectant mothers I have known, I have come to believe that every baby is wanted.

For the first three months of pregnancy, there is always some extra fatigue.

'I simply can't finish making the bed in the morning,' one patient said to me.

'You mean it bothers you to bend over?' I asked.

'Oh, no. It's too inviting. I just crawl in!' she replied.

Another lamented, telling of a posh dinner party she had looked forward to for weeks, 'There I was beside the handsomest guest of honour I've ever seen. He was so interesting too. But I couldn't help it. I fell asleep at the table!'

Every pregnant woman should have at least two hours rest after lunch – with her feet up, and sleeping if possible.

In the first three months her body needs this rest to help adjust to the pregnancy. During these months, when miscarriage is most likely, avoiding overactivity and getting regular extra rest are two important ground rules.

Sally, an energetic young woman with her hockey champion days not far behind her, was in more exuberant health and spirits than ever when she became pregnant six months after her marriage. Enthusiastically she began to plan for the change in her life. This included moving to a new apartment and taking a long automobile trip with her husband, 'because I don't know when I'll be able to go with him on his trips again after the baby comes'. In the hospital, where we saved her from a miscarriage after a nip-and-tuck few days, she admitted she had known she was supposed to be taking extra rest, but she 'never got around to it'. I was exasperated to find she had also continued going horseback riding a couple of times a week.

Most patients go to the other extreme, however. Sometimes I wonder if some aren't so scared of having a miscarriage that they bring it on. It's hard to get across the idea that if you take reasonable care of yourself, there's no call to anticipate a miscarriage; and that if you have one, that doesn't necessarily mean you'll have another. About thirty per cent of all pregnancies end in miscarriage, but Nature knows what she's doing, for nearly three-quarters of these are due to a malformed egg.

After a miscarriage, a woman will feel fatigued and depressed. It's discouraging not to accomplish what you set out to do. I can tell you her doctor feels sad, too. I think both patient and doctor feel frustration and grief, but neither should ever feel regret.

In the last three months, the pregnant woman should be storing up energy for labour. Never forget, labour is appropriately named. For a few hours a woman has a full-time job, calling for all the resources her body can muster. I tell my patients *never* to short cut on the afternoon rest after the sixth month. Actually this may be the only way to get enough sleep at this stage of the game. General discomfort and need for frequent trips to the bathroom often keep a mother-to-be restless and wakeful at night. If she happens to be a stomach sleeper she has an additional frustration.

There's a kind of lull for a pregnant woman in the middle three months. She has more energy. Since these are the best months for working, I have often thought maternity leaves could fit in with nature better than they do. It would be far better for a girl to have leave from her job for the first and last three months than to start it just as she's getting adjusted to pregnancy and beginning to feel more energetic.

Some girls, like Jane, a career girl patient of mine, want to stay on the job throughout pregnancy. Jane and I worked out four energy-saving rules which she came to appreciate more and more as time went on: First, get more night-time sleep. (She changed her bedtime from eleven-thirty to ten-thirty during the week, went out only on evenings when she could sleep an hour or two later the next morning.) Second, split the evening household chores. (Her husband took over all evening dish-washing.) Third, cut down on work in the last three months. (She arranged to work shorter hours, take fewer assignments.) Fourth, in the first and last three months, do a minimum of household work and party-giving or party-going.

Even with all the reassurance and warning I dispense, some patients skip the extra rest, for what seem to be awfully good reasons. They simply *have* to finish their Christmas shopping, for instance. Every year at least one of my patients finishes her shopping all right, but ends up spending Christmas in bed surrounded by Kleenex and aspirin. If it hadn't been a cold, it would have been something else. The human body has a wondrous way of waging its own advance-guard action against overtiredness.

The woman in her third, fourth or fifth pregnancy doesn't have to be impressed with the need for rest. She can hardly wait to have her baby because it will mean a week in bed, which is her idea of a vacation. All she wants is a *chance* to get daily rest. To do it, though, she has to be wily and realistic—wily enough to seize the moment when the older children are at school and the younger ones are napping, realistic enough to put a pillow over the phone and make up her mind not to answer the doorbell. Deciding what to let slide is an art to be mastered by every woman of modern times; the woman pregnant with her sixth baby must be a genius in this department!

A hidden cause of fatigue in pregnancy is the stress of fear. For all its naturalness, having a baby is an awesome thing. Mixed with the awe is some fear – of one's body, of one's ability to have a baby. Bringing new life rouses fear of death. Apprehension about labour and delivery is often not so much dread of pain but, as one patient expressed it, 'being afraid I'll make a fool of myself'. Lastly, there is the fear of having an abnormal baby. There is something about a young woman's pregnancy that primes the pump of old wives' tales. A wealth of new ones are added every generation to all the old hoary ones.

I go on the theory that a doctor's job is to take over, for about a year. It takes just about that to see it through. Particularly with her first baby, a young mother has fears of various sorts until the baby actually comes, proves to be healthy, and attains the age of three months.

'Don't trust yourself or anyone else,' I say flatly to my patients. 'Ask me instead. I'm taking over while you go through this. When the time comes, I'll give yourself back to you!'

It takes from six to twelve weeks to get used to having a baby around. At the six weeks' check-up time, some women have mastered this task and are squared away. Another type shows up dead tired, circles under her eyes, hair uncombed; she's going to need the full three months to get life under control. For the occasional young mother who still hasn't overcome extreme fatigue in this time, special help is in order.

Incidentally, never underestimate the fatigue of a young father. He has to learn to do a lot of new things. For instance, if he doesn't already know how to cook, he'd better learn. He must know how to care for his wife and get ready to look after a baby. It can be rather difficult for him during pregnancy when his wife is not able to have intercourse, although in all the years I have practised medicine I have never heard a wife complain of her husband's attitude towards her during her pregnancy. I have always felt that during that period men adhere to a certain standard of behaviour.

Sometimes even when his wife is ready to resume their sex life six weeks after the baby's birth, a husband is too tired. The anxiety of the whole experience may weigh heavily on him. Add to this the many incidents—sometimes some of them pretty subtle – in the first weeks of the baby's life that keep reminding the father of his displacement as kingpin. Most rise manfully to the situation's demands, but none should be surprised if he feels more tired than usual.

The third and last time a woman experiences great endocrine change is at the menopause. Literally, this is adolescence in reverse – the ending of the cyclic life.

No one knows exactly when the menopause starts; no

one knows exactly when it finishes. There is no known test to prove that a woman is in the menopause. For the sake of my patients' peace of mind, I have often wished we had something like the 'rabbit test' for pregnancy. So far as we know, animals don't have menopause, so they are no help to us.

I have wished, too, that I could be specific enough to say to a patient, 'You are going to start menopause when you are forty-four. You will have one bad year at forty-six. By the time you are forty-eight, it will be over and you will be fine.' But you can't put your finger on the timing of it any more than you can say adolescence begins and ends at certain ages.

My experience is that menopause generally starts in the middle forties, reaches its peak in about two years and is over at fifty. I have known patients who began in the thirties, or as late as fifty-seven, but these were unusual instances. Women live through it first and realize the timing of different stages later.

My patients who got through menopause before or after their children were at the peak of adolescence have thanked their lucky stars. Others, whose timing wasn't favourable, have had a rare experience. One of these patients had twin daughters, who seemed to be fairly mild and well-mannered, as adolescents go; to their mother, who confessed to me that some days she felt she lived 'on the razoredge of doom', they were overwhelming.

Another patient in menopause told me shamefacedly, 'I hate myself for it, but my kids drive me crazy. I know the pin-curl, skin-lotion days will pass and it's just a phase, but I can't stand the way they look when they come to the table. So I blow my top, and the next thing I know they're in their room studying the siren techniques most likely to be successful with the boys at school.'

Another mother had patiently worked for years helping her child who was a slow learner. When she realized that menopause was reducing her store of patience, she very sensibly arranged for the youngster, by then a teenager, to have special training in a day school.

The onset and tapering-off of both adolescence and menopause is gradual. Mother Nature usually approaches her changes in a quite leisurely fashion. One cheerful thought a woman has to hang on to in this period of transition is that it will end. Not only that, the best years of her life are ahead.

Drastic changes in amounts of available energy occur from day to day during menopause – sometimes even from one hour of the day to another. These changes vary according to the metabolic state of the body, which in turn depends on the stress under which the body is functioning. In recent years research has been carried on to try to determine the varying quantities of hormones put out during menopause and the kind of interaction among different hormones, but we do not yet know a great deal about it.

Along with fluctuations in energy, there are shifts in emotional balance. Remember adolescence? Remember pregnancy? It's the same story. The glands are changing and the nervous system, which is usually in control of the whole operation, is not quite up to scratch in its correlating job. This is what makes you unable to remember the title of the book you finished reading yesterday or the name of the author; why you may, like one friend of mine, patiently stuff the teapot with the tea cosy instead of the teabags. You may find yourself in tears because the jelly won't jell or you can't find your other bedroom slipper. Cheer up, you're having a bad day. Tomorrow will probably be better.

It has always seemed to me too bad that at such a trying time, women should have to cope with embarrassing symptoms like flushing and unexpected haemorrhages. I'm glad that today we have pills to help alleviate the flushing, though women should remember they are for true flushing. Those who burn out of pure nervousness are not helped.

It is true that while some women have scanty periods of menstruation months apart, others have heavier periods occurring quite close together. Both are normal more often than not, but a woman should keep precise records of irregular bleeding and report them to her doctor.

Women the world over have the same experience at menopause. Wherever they live, they go through it in exactly the same way. At international medical meetings, I am interested to see that identical problems are described in papers given by doctors from all parts of the world. The differences come out in the way people feel about a particular symptom. All women are tired, but in one country they are alarmed because fatigue cuts down on their efficiency and in another they are upset because it makes them temporarily indifferent to a sex life.

The first thing to do about menopause is to understand it, just as the first thing to do about your daughter's adolescence is to understand it – and help her to understand it.

Establish the fact in your mind that the most significant thing about the menopause is the glandular change taking place, and that this, because of the deep involvement of your metabolic patterns, will affect the amount of energy you will have available from day to day. Soon you will begin to be aware that you are having a bad day or a good day, and that it's nothing to worry about. Then you will plan accordingly.

'Well,' you will say to yourself, 'this is one of those days. I have no energy. I feel awful. I don't want to go out or do anything. I wish I had stayed in bed,' or 'This is a good day. This is the day to get that chore done.'

Those good days can get you in trouble, there's no doubt about that. This is one of the funniest aspects of the menopause, if you can see it that way. You agree, on a good day of course, to do all sorts of things – have the family for Thanksgiving, entertain the club, chauffeur a carful of people on an all-day swim and picnic. Come the day and it happens to be a bad one. You can't decide what to wear or what to have to eat. You don't feel competent to drive the car. You take a jaundiced view of seeing even your best friend, let alone a group of people youll' have to play hostess to, or at least talk to.

After a while you learn, though. On those good days, you can do more, but you don't use up all your week's quota of energy in planning a party that you're not going to be able to carry out without panic. You plan parties for fewer people, or arrange for more help. You keep your social life, but keep it flexible and informal. Be prepared to conserve energy. But make up your mind that if there's nothing else to do about it, you'll see it through.

Where women in menopause make their mistake is in not understanding what they need. My prescription calls for recreation, laughter, stimulation and extra rest. Given these, a woman can get on with it, enjoying the good days, taking the bad days in her stride. When she wakes up feeling like something the cat dragged in, she should do what she absolutely must, then do something she likes to do. Go shopping or go to the movies. If she has to go to work, she should try to make it as much of a 'coasting' day as she can and promise herself that to-night she will do something that really appeals to her.

You might not believe it, but I have known women to discover an entirely new career or engrossing hobby because they kept their eyes open for something that would brighten up those tired, dejected days. One of my patients who took her child to painting class every week stayed to watch one day simply because she was too tired and dispirited to get going again. She got so interested, she decided to try her hand at it while she was waiting, though she hardly knew which end of the brush to use. In no time she had joined a painting class of her own, and eventually turned out very creditable work.

Another patient decided on a good day to capitalize on the bad days by writing humorous sketches about them. Later she developed some of these into stories which she was able to place in women's magazines. A new career may await still another patient who writes poems when she can't sleep at night, if she ever can bring herself to submit them for editorial scrutiny!

To combat fatigue, an agenda is in order. My own estimate is that on an average a woman has about eighty per cent of her normal energy and efficiency during her menopause years. This may vary from ninety per cent on one day to ten per cent on another.

Plan on that. Make sure you have a certain amount of time during the day that is your own. When your emotional tone is low and dreary, do not drive yourself through a too-rigorous schedule. Do what you can. If you try too hard to discipline yourself, 'pull yourself together', you fall apart. If you are a 'tired businesswoman' you need refreshment of mind and light-hearted laughter. Get it into your programme for the week.

Both the teen-age youngster and the middle-aged woman need intelligent understanding from family and friends. But the worst thing in the world for a menopausing woman is sympathy. It may seem as though she wants it, but actually she'd rather be taken out to dinner.

In any case, a woman in menopause should not compare her energy to that of women in other age brackets.

c

The woman who complains. 'My mother works rings around me and she's in her sixties,' is probably in her own tired forties. She will be doing the same as her mother when *she* is sixty.

An understanding of one's own frailties and a sense of humour are the two most important foundations, in this period of life as in all others. If you are fortunate enough to be surrounded by love and affection, don't drain it dry, but go out to it, give to it.

A woman in adolescence, in the prenatal period, in menopause, has this experience over and over again: energy just disappears; she feels exhausted. This is normal for a woman, just as normal as being interested in the fall fashions or wanting to try out a new recipe. It's part of the female heritage. Alas, 'tis her frailty, not she!

6

A Time to be Born and a Time to Die

THERE IS a natural order of life, and in this order of things we must live. A time to be born and a time to die; a time for being young and helpless and a time for growing up; a time for falling in love; a time for growing older. We cannot change this any more than we can change the passage of time itself.

Part of the secret in mastering the fatigue problem is knowing and accepting Nature's timing. I speak not only of the laws of physiological growth and biological development. Life inevitably brings sorrow, suffering, joy, contentment, struggle, achievement and disappointment. There is a time for each of these. We have the choice between accepting them in faith – faith in life as a whole – or fighting them in bitterness and loneliness. Truly he who tries to 'save his life' shall lose it.

Wisdom comes from the awareness of timing, recognition of change, and knowledge of one's own limitations.

True, the clamour of modern life sometimes obscures that deeply personal sense of rhythm and timing in our lives. It gets lost in the blare of radio and television, the whirring of labour-saving devices, the urgent beep of the car waiting at the door, the insistent ring of the telephone. But we must keep close to the murmur of that inner melody that tells us who we are and what we are about; otherwise we will be pushed here and there on ceaseless waves of life which get us nowhere.

Several years ago a Canadian educator wrote that modern education in my country was asking too little of our children. I realized I had long thought our aims for our children (except those for their economic security) were too low. We protect them from the challenge of life, from the knowledge that there is a law of cause and effect – that there are consequences for each deed we perform, for each decision we act on. We do not encourage them to adventure, to explore. We deny them the thrill of having a brand-new idea, or recognizing those of others.

Obstacles, challenges, inspiration – these are natural parts of life. Protecting children and adolescents from them weakens the fibres which will have to stand up to the inevitable sorrow and tragedy of life.

Most parents want to feel that their children arrive at good choices, preferably under their own steam. But from my observation, they mistakenly try to keep the decision-making atmosphere free of struggle. The young daughter of a patient of mine recently decided to continue college study in her home town after seriously considering transfer to a university in another part of the country. During the whole period in which she was making up her mind, the fact that the move would place a heavy expense upon her parents was never discussed.

There is a time for realizing one can't do something

because one can't afford it. My patient was happy that her daughter had made a choice without being confronted with this struggle. I think the parents denied her a useful experience which would help when she comes to make another difficult decision. I feel strongly that youngsters should learn that life is a struggle while they are still bolstered by the security of their own homes.

The teens are the time to learn – to learn about life, about oneself, about love. And it is the time to learn how to earn a living. Though today's teen-ager has many sources of guidance – school, church, clubs – he should be able to turn to his own parents for his greatest need, what we might call 'leadership'. The best place to learn about life is at home.

Because teen-agers of today appear to be sophisticated, they are often credited with being more emotionally mature than they really are. They may know more facts, have a descriptive vocabulary, and be more knowledgeable about biology than the teen-agers of ten or twenty years ago. But they have less responsibility, more protection and security – and show it! They accustom themselves to conformity and take every means of escape in order to avoid making a hard, tough decision. Why do fifteen-year-olds go steady? They can't take a chance on being wallflowers, on not having a date for a dance.

'I hate being fifteen,' a pretty youngster confided to me as she poured out her feelings about a dilemma which included a devoted steady and a set of disapproving parents. 'Everything is so confused.'

She is so right! For the fifteen-year-old, the confusion is so real you can cut it with a knife. I wouldn't want to be fifteen again for anything in the world. But I'm not sure I'd want to be the mother of a fifteen-year-old either! There's no easy way to live through an age of change.

As I told my young friend, the thing to do is live the age one is in. Now is the time for her to get an adequate education, not only a technical one which will give her a vocation, but the chance to develop mind and spirit as well. In the school years there are so many other things to do besides dating and making sure you have a bid to the dance.

A person this young must let go of the feeling of being important to only one person. There will come a time when she will be so engrossed in a man that she will want to have lunch with him, spend the evening with him, have him phone to say good night. It is a beautiful experience, and important that it happen sometime. But it cannot happen and survive at fifteen.

The very next day after this conversation, I was approached by an eighteen-year-old who had been going steady for two years. Her problem was that her boy friend, 'a wonderful person', was still terribly serious about her. Her feelings just weren't the same, but she didn't want to hurt him.

It was so understandable. No one wants to hurt a person she likes and respects. But this is a hazard of the strict ground rules of going steady. The truth is that, for young people of this age, if new interests become more important so that earlier ties are broken, then that is the way life should go. If there is anything real in the relationship, it will survive the new interests and grow stronger.

Another thing I think young people overlook is that if two people have a deep affection for each other, even if it does not grow into love, they will never lose each other. A genuine friendship is one of life's most precious gifts.

We should not lose sight of the fact that despite superficial sophistications and the rise and fall of fads in behaviour, the basic needs of the teen-ager are the same as they always were. They need security in their homes and a belief that they belong. This is how they find the inner security that will carry them through their adult years. At the same time they must have enough freedom to wean themselves gradually from too close family life. They are like beginning swimmers who need to touch bottom now and then to make sure it is really there.

A teen-ager's insecurity arises from his rapid physical and emotional growth. Today he may revert to childhood habits. Tomorrow he may advance to adult thinking and behaviour. Both days he needs a good steady reliable centre of operations.

A sense of responsibility and a wish to share should flow from the experience of teen-age. Specifically, teen-age is the time to develop responsibility to education, to the value of money, to the use of time, to an appreciation of inevitability of action and reaction. I have said that today's crop of teen-agers tend to be less responsible than former generations. I believe our way of life is partly to blame. Families on wheels make for fluid communities in which people either don't put down their roots, or don't put them down very far. Many more people live in apartments, which means less responsibility for everyone, including young people. Looser community ties means that community opinion is not so powerful as a shaper of standards for behaviour.

Today women need all the education they can get. Most girls will work for a living, if not all their lives, at least in three time spans – until they marry, for a while after they marry until they begin their families, and again when their families are grown. Whether or not they work for money, they will be called upon to do volunteer work, to serve on boards and committees. Better yet, they will actively seek to work in their church and community groups. Now that an education is available to her, a woman should get the best one she can, the one most suited to her talents and abilities.

I look forward to the day when all women are better educated when young. Perhaps then there will be no more lonely, bored, dreary, middle-aged women who don't know what to do with themselves when their children are grown.

Young people sometimes try to hurry the rhythm of life. They want to move into adult responsibilities before they are ready. In fact, often it seems to me that the less ready, the more eager they are to plunge ahead! Not long ago a sixteen-year-old girl asked my advice.

For three years she had been caring for her younger brothers and sisters because both of her parents worked. She was in a kicking-over-the-traces mood, wanting to leave school and get a job, leave home and take an apartment with friends.

'I want dates with no kids around,' she told me, 'I want money of my own to buy some decent clothes. It's time my ten-year-old sister took over at home.'

Her feelings were legitimate, her wants understandable. But she had lost sight of the fact that the plans she was making would affect the rest of her life.

'It is essential that you get as good an education as you can,' I told her. 'This is not just for today, but for ten or fifteen years from now when it may not be so easy to get a job.'

Another strong feeling I had was that the big changes she proposed to make are the kind that have to be timed. Her little sister would need help in learning to assume responsibility for the younger children. And for her own sake, she should take at least a year to work towards departure from the family group.

'Don't ever cut your roots from your family suddenly,' was my advice to her, 'especially when there is confusion of your ideas about why you are doing it. The roots you put down are important to your whole life. You must never cut them off because of your desire to be free for the happiness of the moment. You are really preparing yourself for the kind of life you're going to live for the next seventy years, whether it seems that way to you or not.'

Fortunately we can get back in step with the rhythm of life, if we have the wit to see we've gotten off beat. We are always doing this in small ways. We resolve to spend more time at home, stick to a budget, pay more attention to personal appearance, plan meals more carefully.

I believe adults have responsibility to the young, not only to help them with timing but help them regain it when necessary. There's no point in saying, 'Well, she's only fifteen but she's gone and gotten married and now she's going to have a baby. She's carved out her life.' If she's missed a turn or taken a curve too fast, the adults in her life can try to help her grow as much as possible in the normal pattern.

I talked with just such a child wife recently. No fifteen-year-old has the qualifications of a mother, I told her. Children have a right to a mother who has some education and experience of life, some maturity. I suggested that she get to work and learn some more, go back to school.

She was astonished. 'Go back to school? Why, I'm going to have a baby.'

'Having a baby doesn't stop life,' I said. 'Go to night school. Learn to type, or to cook, but learn something. Don't just sit home and wait for your baby. Be able to do something, even if it's to cook three good meals a day.'

She sparked to that. I think it was the first time she'd felt any real responsibility to be a person.

It is a very common experience for me to see girls and

even young women who appear to feel that being in love with someone who loves them and wanting to get married and have a home is the be-all and end-all of life. Like my young friend, they have not had a glimmer that there is something more in the life of the mind than what has been presented to them in their high school classes.

There is a time to learn about love, to learn about sex and its place in the scheme of things.

Sex life does not begin with marriage. For any human being, it begins with the waking up to the powerful force of life each of us has within us. We have a sense of being drawn into a new world, of embarking upon the most miraculous adventure of life.

In my home town there was a little boy, red-haired and freckled. One day after school he asked if he could carry my books home for me. We always walked home together, but up to this point I had always carried my own books, and sometimes his too. On this day suddenly the whole pattern of life turned upside down. If the world had opened up at my feet and begun spouting lava, I would not have been more astounded. Life would never be so secure again for me. I had sensed the power of being a woman.

Sex is power. Just being male and female has power attached to it. You have to do something about it. You can't get rid of it. From this moment of self-discovery, you know you have this powerful something within you. And you retain it. One thing women and men forget is that marriage – going into a church and making a pledge in good faith – has no magic effect upon this potential power. They are still male and female. They still have the responsibility for seeing to it that the power does not get out of hand.

There are three reactions to this discovery. Some like to use it for all it's worth, literally to find out what they can get out of it. Some, overwhelmed by the insecurity of the experience, decide they don't like it and will stay away from it, deny it and avoid it. The intelligent, well-adjusted boys and girls decide they like it but know they must respect it.

The power of sex goes all through life. A person must go out to meet it and make it his own. A pale spinster with no vitality, unloved and unloving, is paying a price for her fear. So is the bachelor who remains attached to his mother.

On winter evenings, as I drive across a bridge which spans a ravine on my way home, sometimes I see the lights go on all at once for miles to my right and left. It never fails to give me a renewed awe at the enormous power of electricity. Sex is like that. It has the potential for wonderful illumination – and for blinding destruction. It must be respected. A young person who does not know this – or believe it – is not yet out of the ABC class in the facts of life. One of the wisest of old sayings is, 'It isn't what you've got but what you do with it, that counts.'

There is a time for marrying. It is not when all your friends are getting married and you think you'd better seize the moment and the handiest prospect. It is not the minute two young people are able to support each other. And it is not simply when they have gone steady for three years, each avoiding all other opportunities to date other boys and girls. It is when they are grown up enough to know what the responsibilities of marriage are and to be able to assume them. It is when they have experienced love, when they know the difference between love and physical attraction. The feeling of needing the other person in order to feel like a complete human being is part of it. So is the willingness to pool their lives, without reservation, come what may – with some knowledge of what may come!

The son of a patient of mine married, at nineteen, a girl he had gone steady with for three years. All seemed to go well with the marriage for about two years. They had a beautiful baby, the husband progressed in his job, they were saving money for a home. Suddenly he became enamoured of a girl in his office.

'He comes right out and says he never knew what it was to be in love before,' my patient told me, her distress for the young couple bringing tears to her eyes.

'He probably never did,' I answered. 'His wife is the only girl he ever dated, isn't she?'

'Yes,' she sighed. 'They were so sweet together. Just seemed made for each other.'

'Perhaps it will work out eventually, then,' I said, but inwardly I wondered for the thousandth time what young people and their parents can be thinking of when they take such unrealistic views about marriage.

Increased financial security has made it possible for

many young people to marry earlier than they might have. Because our civilization is so oriented to economic security, both young people and their parents are too prone to judge readiness for marriage in terms of what two pay cheques add up to. In most cases I am wary of the two-income marriage, the one where the wife must go on working in order for the young couple to live. Women should not work just to provide income. They should work because they get satisfaction from doing something they do well. Working for money just to perpetuate life can turn into a life sentence, with the wife becoming an adjunct to her husband's work. A married woman's job should be part of a plan worked out in a partnership aimed towards mutual goals.

Deep within each of us there is the sure knowledge of the right timing of life experiences for us. If we do not know ourselves well enough to recognize it, the knowledge may come to us in roundabout ways.

I remember a seventeen-year-old who came in to me for a premarital examination. She was normal in every way, but her whole body showed what a state of tension she was in. She admitted to feeling unusually tired.

'Perhaps it would be wise to postpone your marriage until you're a bit more relaxed and rested,' I said. 'There's plenty of time.'

She burst into tears.

'I can't,' she said. 'I have to go through with it.'

She certainly wasn't pregnant; my examination had shown that.

'Can you tell me why?' I asked gently.

'My mother and father have set their hearts on this boy. He's like a member of the family already. And I've gone with him for three years. I'm afraid if I don't hurry and get through with it, I'll do something terrible, like run away or something.'

I was appalled. She was like a drowning person. Everything in her heart told her not to take this step at this time, but she was too young and too frail in spirit to follow her own inner advice without the support of her parents. Her mother, whom I saw later, had not realized how unsure her daughter was. The marriage was postponed, I was happy to learn.

This youngster had started going steady because it seems to be a custom – to my mind, not a very good one. It's kind of an insurance; girls know they will always have a date, and boys find it convenient and less expensive. Thanks to this comfortable arrangement, neither has to make any effort to learn to handle a new situation or adapt to a new personality. They settle into this pattern so completely sometimes that they find they can't even dance with other partners. They know one another's minds and opinions as well as the lyrics of their favourite hit tunes. They become fixtures in each other's homes.

It's wonderful for boys and girls to be good friends. But marriage for a girl who has gone steady with one boy since she came of dating age will be no adventure. It will just be carrying on the same pattern with a different round of tasks. How can she be expected to have the stamina and wisdom to make a husband happy by giving herself completely? Let's face it, how will she have the wit to withstand the beguiling of another man's desire?

If a young person knows too little about herself and what she wants and what life really is, it is, I believe, the job of adults to help her be more adventurous. It isn't enough that these young women put on the trappings of adulthood: a 'Mrs' in front of a name, a ring on a finger. They should have more chance to learn what life is about – the struggle of learning about themselves in relation to other people, the effort and the adjustment on which all true happiness and all true marriages are based.

Parents' goal for their daughters should not be just the fact of marriage. If a couple are determined that their daughter shall have an adequate education, knowledge of life and an ability to love, their reward will be an inner contentment as they watch their daughter walk through life with dignity and grace.

There is a time for growing older.

There is no tiredness quite like the fatigue that comes from fighting age. The passing years and what they do to the human body add up to something as inevitable and fundamental as the facts of life. Yet you can't imagine the numbers of people who pit their precious energies against this inexorable force, instead of co-operating with it. Many of my patients who ask, 'Why am I so tired?' have to admit finally that they are trying to fight this losing battle every day of their lives.

If you are born a female, a female you will be to the end of your days. And it is just as inescapable that at the end of forty years, you are going to be forty, look like forty, and – if you are wise – act like it!

It's natural to bemoan the appearance of greying hair and wrinkles in the neck, but resistance and panic are no ways to solve the problem. The woman who goes haywire and has 'one last fling' to alleviate her distress about the changes age is bringing about might better have gotten it out of her system by seeing a couple of torrid movies. Putting up this kind of fight may bring real tragedy to a woman and those she loves. I well remember two women who took out their panic by competing with their young daughters.

In one case, both mother and daughter were extraordinarily beautiful. Far from being proud of this lovely miniature of herself, the mother became over-critical, nagging and spiteful. The daughter, in her unhappiness, grew to be reckless and undiscriminating in her choice of companions, and finally ran away from home to make a poor marriage.

The daughter of the other woman was much less attractive than her mother. Unable to accept the child's rather homely appearance, as well as her own advancing years, the woman got herself invited to the younger crowd's parties – under the guise of 'helping Karen out with her social life'. Her behaviour made her appear a fool. Ashamed and suffering, the girl began to drink and became an alcoholic.

Personally, I think some things about growing older

D

are funny; others are wonderful. There is something especially attractive and interesting about a middle-aged or older woman who has lived fully, growing in wisdom and the ability to love as she went along.

One very droll thing about a woman is that she combats age by making every conceivable change in her face and hair-do, and all the time she has a fine roll around the middle, which is where age really shows.

The thing we really ought to fear and combat about age is its rigidity. We love the flexibility of youth. That doesn't necessarily have to disappear with age.

I can understand the loneliness of the woman whose children are married and gone, whose husband has died. I can understand the fears of the woman who faces living the rest of her life with a chronic illness or handicap, or who must enter the working world for the first time late in life in order to earn a living. I can sympathize with the single woman who must come face to face with the fact that she will probably not be truly loved and desired by a mate and certainly will have no children. My heart aches for the married woman who has wanted a child so badly and now the years have run out.

But the women who spend their energy grappling fiercely with such an inevitable force as time itself, I do not understand.

And for those who must cope with real problems brought about by life, the years and circumstances, I say this: that heartbreak can be healed, and there is always a need for love and affection among those who are near and dear to us.

I believe the most important things to women of any age are affection, being needed, a sense of achievement, and faith in the whole of life. The last we can gain for ourselves as we come to know that any aspect of life, any phase of it, may fall short of our dreams and aspirations at some time. And there is a blessed wonder about reaching an age when at last we know what we are, and we feel true maturity growing within us. There is power in this realization; it frees us to know what we can do, what kind of people we can be, what we can put into life.

'Getting older isn't so bad,' a patient said to me. 'I get a kick out of the youngsters' plans for after college, getting married, and so on. And I have more time than I ever had to spend with my husband. We laugh at each other a little, but we're really looking forward to having grandchildren too.'

As for menopause, that's just a transition stage. One thing I hope I accomplished in my first book was to make people laugh at this stage, which is really quite comical, even though difficult. And so well worth while just getting through, too! I have said often and still say that the lovely fifties bring a sense of inner vigour and well-being, a sense that life is for living and this is the time to do it. It incenses me that women, with all their fine assets, fall for this false idea that when youth begins to go, life isn't worth living. When they yield to fright, and struggle against age, they open themselves to the kind of fatigue which keeps them from ever lighting up over anything.

A woman who has succeeded in making herself look younger than she is has a special hazard. Every time she looks at herself in the mirror, she puts herself in competition with her real age all over again. This woman is quite likely to be the one, too, who prides herself on being a sister or comrade to her children. I don't know of any worse mistake modern parents can make. As Noel Coward puts it in his witty song, 'What's going to happen to the children when there aren't any more grownups?'

Women whose greatest ambition is to be young and decorative are indeed fighting a losing battle. It takes a lot of time out of anybody's schedule. And there is nothing so fatiguing as to fight against nature. Nature always wins.

There is a time for everything. Each decade in a woman's life is different. If she lives each to its fullest, and meets each with acceptance, she grows in grace and happiness.

7

Common Sense and Calories

TAKE IT for granted that good energy production goes hand-in-hand with a good state of nutrition. What food is required by the human energy-production plant, and when, and how much? Food experts differ. So do the requirements of individuals. Nutrition has a lot to do with fatigue, but there's nothing mysterious about it. It's just a matter of common sense.

A great many people assume that a certain intake of calories at stated intervals each day is essential to produce a required amount of energy. In the long run we do need a certain caloric intake over a certain period, but this is not necessarily true of the short haul. If you feel tired and your stomach is empty, you may be feeling the need of a rest period rather than the need for calories. Many people have learned that just sitting down and having a cup of black coffee gives them a new lease on life, especially if time is taken off from work to do it.

Some years ago, a study was made of a group of soldiers who were tired in the middle of the morning. A large proportion of them were found to have a low concentration of sugar in their blood. At first it seemed that the lack of glucose in the blood was the cause of fatigue. Then an equal number of energetic, unfatigued soldiers were tested. They had the same low concentration of sugar. It had to be concluded that the fatigue of the first group was not due to an inadequate amount of calories taken in the last few hours before fatigue overtook them.

Inadequate diet over a long period of time is another question entirely. A poor state of nutrition can undoubtedly cause fatigue, but this is not common in our part of the world. The hard working, underfed coolie in the East subsists on food deficient in calories as well as essential vitamins and minerals. This is a far cry from the diet of the average Canadian and American.

Among our new Canadians, there are many who have undergone great suffering in Europe, including periods of near starvation. I have treated women of this group who cannot conceive a child because their general physical condition does not seem to allow it. Even so, an adequate diet, rest and care can usually give these patients confidence and hope in a matter of months.

Of course doctors do see cases of malnutrition. Most often these are people who have replaced their food by drink, or continued for a long period on a faddish diet. Now and then there will be a patient who has developed an emotional reaction against food; these cases are rare except among alcoholics and patients on such fixed diets as those for diabetics.

Just as our metabolisms differ, our food requirements differ. Some people feel they need a good breakfast if they are going to do a good morning's work. Others can't work well after a big meal, and want only coffee and orange juice for breakfast because they get their best work done before the first meal of the day. In our society eating three meals a day is the normal pattern, but there's nothing against going without breakfast or lunch as long as the stomach and digestive tract are not stirred up with strong coffee or some other stimulating beverage.

We cannot always be hungry at mealtime. Sometimes we are so absorbed or involved by other things that food isn't so alluring, for the moment. This is perfectly normal. Most of us overeat at times, too, and there is nothing wrong with that, either. The thing to remember is that the total amount of food taken in day by day should be in proportion to the amount of physical work we do. Because we live in a society of abundance and many of us lead comparatively sedentary lives, this calls for restraint in eating for most of us.

There is no special diet to prevent fatigue. So far, none of the fad diets making this claim have really worked. Food faddists are thought by some psychiatrists to be suffering from emotional illness. Certainly many of them are naïve; they believe what they want to believe without very good evidence of the truth of their assumptions. Occasionally a doctor will find that a patient has done real, perhaps irreparable, harm to herself by following a fad diet. I remember a woman who had developed an anaemia which no amount of iron or liver could really correct in months, even years. But on the whole, food faddists probably do themselves more harm by their way of thinking and behaving than by concentrating on some foods and ignoring others.

There is no better diet, ordinarily, than the one a person has been eating for the last ten, twenty or thirty years. If this is proving to be dangerous because she is putting on extra weight, the answer is to cut it in half or two thirds. Certainly it is not to change to some bizarre menu which makes one either a martyr or a fool and tends to disrupt the usual eating habits of the family or group to which she belongs.

Dieting or putting too much importance on what we eat or don't eat reminds us three times a day of the physical defect we are trying to correct, so most of us don't do it unless we have to. If we must diet, we are happier if we don't make a fetish out of it.

Fatigue certainly results from eating too much, though it's a glorious feeling sometimes to be too full. We do not jump up to do the dishes, rush to write letters or sit inspired at a meeting; we are more apt to feel, if not fatigued, at least relaxed. Sometimes this is a good time to catch a little nap.

Continuous overeating cannot help but furnish us with too much weight to carry around. Although most people put it on an ounce at a time, so that the increase is hardly noticed from week to week, extra weight is tiring in ways a person may not be aware of. It is harder to bend over; it is harder to bend at all. It is harder to take a big breath, and breathing is one of the automatic but continuous bits of work we have to do. Joints wear out much less quickly if they have less work to do. If your family has a tendency to grow arthritic or rheumatic as they grow older, be careful not to add to the work or the leg and back joints by putting on too much weight.

It is important to retain your normal weight in adulthood. Eating the proper amount of food is as essential as getting the proper vitamins into your diet.

Taking off weight suddenly is not a good thing, certainly not the answer to being overweight.

A person who tends to put on weight will never change this basic pattern. She must be prepared to live a life of dietary discipline for ever. A harsh thought, but true!

Let's look at the other side of the energy coin. Patients often ask, 'Should I be taking exercise, and what kind?'

I like to recall the cartoon of the tremendously fat calisthenics director doing his morning radio broadcast, 'One, two, push up, three, four', while lying comfortably in bed.

Some people enjoy starting the day with a few simple exercises, and this may make them feel very much more alert. Others find such shenanigans uninteresting, unsatisfactory and a waste of time. The average person feels better with a little exercise every day, or every other day. But some people can be perfectly healthy without moving out of bed, off the chair, or out of their car.

Exercise should be a recreation, enjoyable for itself, not some kind of price paid for good health. Some people go at it as they would a diet, taking it too seriously and in short spurts. It should be something that can be done easily, conveniently and preferably with friends. Remember when you were young and a game of tennis made you feel healthy and vigorous while scrubbing the kitchen floor made you tired? Probably the two called for about the same amount of exercise and energy.

We lead awfully protected lives in our modern world. But keeping our muscles well trained may be extra insurance for emergencies. A little walking and you'll be better able to run for the bus to make that important appointment. A few push-ups and you can push your own car when it runs out of gas, instead of having to wait for the garage man.

Do not eat to combat fatigue.

Remember that too much weight and too rigid muscles are two of our greatest enemies.

Make energy, then use it. Health is not an end in itself, but a good physique and lots of energy help make for a full and happy life.

8

Secrets of Happy Family Life

MOST MOTHERS of young children work too much and do not rest enough. The same goes for mothers of any age children who try to run a home with one hand and a job with the other. Too often the results are strained family relations. Sometimes fatigue boils over into serious physical or mental problems for the woman.

The fatigue of a mother is the single most important element in any family's emotional well-being. If the mother is too tired, she can't be judicious in the treatment and discipline of her children, or give the proper love and attention to her husband. She suffers and so does her family. The emotional tone of their family life becomes dull, apathetic, inconsistent and irritable.

A mother's fatigue permeates family life in a thousand small ways.

Recently I listened to a tape recording of a group of high-school children discussing family relations. Repeatedly, the youngsters said they wished mothers would 'be calm and listen'. I was particularly struck with this, as I know it is impossible for a fatigued mother to be calm. It takes energy to be calm when things are going all wrong. Another complaint was that mothers keep sending children to the store numerous times a day. It was evident to me that such mothers are tired, and so they are disorganized and forgetful. They send the child to the store and then want something else when he gets home. The child is upset. Dinner is upset. Everything is upset.

The family situations which breed exhausting stresses for a mother are many. Only a few are truly difficult to straighten out. Where there are too many small children, where there is long-term illness or some member of the family is mentally disturbed, the problem may be serious. A lesser kind of fatigue may arise from the constant irritation or frustration of having people outside the immediate family in the house. A special kind of fatigue follows childbirth. Because this may never be understood by the mother (and thus may never be relieved), it can condition the family life for ever, perhaps affecting the mother's feelings about having another child.

After three decades of watching patients come through my office, I have decided there's a predictable pattern of fatigue among mothers who stay at home with their children.

Take Alice, a nice girl who has just had her first baby and is feeling that special tiredness. Like many a new mother before her, Alice felt her first week with the baby at home was a devastating experience, for all the joy the baby's coming brought. She says she's exhausted, but she isn't really; exhaustion takes longer than that. But she *is* fatigued. She's in a stage of adapting to caring for her baby. By the end of three months she may feel tired at the end of the day, but the fatigue she feels now will be gone. Her adaptation will have been completed; her metabolism will be back to normal.

Barbara comes in next. Her first baby is two now, and she's in for a check up after having her second. Barbara complains of pain in her lower back. She doesn't seem to be regaining energy; she feels generally miserable; she's afraid there must be something really wrong. There isn't. She's in fine shape. But she, too, is feeling fatigued by the stress of having two babies to care for. We go over her schedule to make sure she has time for daytime rest, review the rules that will help her adapt to these lively stresses. Can she cut down on some household chores that aren't really necessary? Can her mother come in once a week so she can go out to dinner with her husband? Are there some worries she should talk over frankly with her husband instead of keeping them to herself? Barbara will be all right, too, given a little time.

Close on her heels is Carolyn. Five years ago she went through the first baby stage that Alice is in now. Two years ago she was in the same boat Barbara is in today. Now she's had a third child and has moved into a new echelon of Fatigued Mothers. She's really had it. 'I go to bed tired, I wake up tired, I'm always tired. Don't tell me I'm young and healthy. I know it. But just the same, my mother can do twice as much as I can.' Carolyn has a dozen general complaints. She can't remember when she last had a feeling of well-being. She hints at fears of some kind of terrible disease. If I hadn't lived this pattern over and over with so many young mothers, I might think so myself. But it's the same old thing. Fatigue.

It's the constant, dreary, repetitive limitlessness of work in the home that gets a mother down. It's never done. There's no end to it. It's always with her.

But I have news for Carolyn: her kind of fatigue is easiest to cure. This is going to be a bracer for Barbara and Alice, also, when they get to this stage.

Whether a mother has three children or ten, there are still only twenty-four hours in a day. Then there's another day. The mother who stays home does have some control over how she spends those hours. First of all, the Carolyns must settle for the fact that they have too much to do, that they will not get really rested for several years, that, to some extent, they will always be tired until the children are in school. Then they can put their minds to learning how to control their lives. I know they can; I have seen it happen.

What a child needs most is a lively, lovable mother. If his mother has enough energy to be enthusiastic, enough inner vigour to give off some semblance of a feeling of well-being, a youngster can get along without a lot of other things. Mother's real goal is to see that this need is fulfilled. To do this, she must learn how to keep her inevitable tiredness from getting too far into the fatigue phase.

The woman who is employed outside her home and has a home to look after usually *has* to be at work at a certain time and *has* to get home at a certain time. Her life is scheduled to such an extent that she has much less control over how she plans her day than a woman at home has.

Every woman, whether or not she works, should have a time-energy budget on her own particular 'income' of both. First, make a daily – or weekly – agenda of your duties. Establish the priority items, *including time for sufficient day rest*. Be as ruthless about this as you would about setting aside so much money a week for repairing the roof against the fall rains, taking a vacation next summer away from the office, or paying for the children's education. Keep remembering that a short rest at the time you need it is like money in the bank, only it will pay more dividends.

To do this, you will have to eliminate some non-priority items, shift some activities from priority to non-priority categories, and rearrange or cut down time spent on others. One of my patients who was accustomed to visit her elderly mother on the other side of town each day arranged a schedule with her brother and sister so that each visited twice weekly and phoned on the other days. Another found she got a better balance between energy and social life by making a point of not going out for lunch or afternoon affairs on days when she was going out in the evening with her husband.

Once you begin to examine the items on your list in an objective sort of way, you may find they shift themselves, or even drop out of the list entirely.

You will say, as many of my patients have, that there is not time for rest for a busy housewife, mother or employed woman. If you will use your ingenuity, you can make it.

The mother with small children can get her rest after lunch, while the youngsters are napping. Never mind the ironing which you thought you'd get done while there was peace and quiet. You'll do it better later, even with interruptions and bedlam. If the children go to school, you have more of a choice in picking your time. If nobody gets home till dinner-time, you're in clover!

The working mother has fewer choices about how she will arrange her day, since nearly all jobs have prescribed hours of work. She can get up a little earlier so as to get a more leisurely start on the day, and feel prepared for it. Some of my patients have tried this and found it relieved the work pressure.

Arranging a definite time to rest is a bit more tricky for the working mother, but she must have it. One of my patients found that if she relaxed a half-hour when she first came home, it worked wonders for her.

'It means dinner is a half-hour later,' she told me, 'but the family got used to that. Now I think they like it – probably because I'm better able to carry on a conversation while we eat. That half-hour seems to put things in perspective. It's a bridge between my work life and my home life. After dinner I find myself doing all sorts of things I'd thought of on the way home that should be done but I was too tired to do, like pressing a dress or cleaning out the refrigerator, or listening to my child's music lesson for tomorrow.'

What happens to her, and can happen to any tired

person, is that as she rests she restores herself and her metabolic state.

Timing is important. To combat fatigue successfully, a woman must rest *before* she gets completely tired out each day. Some of my patients have found, also, that taking short rests several times a day worked out better than taking one longer period.

Three basic rules for Operation Fatigue Control are these:

Look upon your rest period as time for yourself. Use it to read, think about or plan something that is important to you as a person.

Make up your mind that some days there is no point in trying to finish anything but the day!

Never delude yourself into thinking that you can make up at night for the rest you did not get all day. Many a well-launched attack on fatigue has foundered upon this mistaken idea.

Changing pace is a helpful technique for happy management of the stresses of life. Changing pace means changing stress. For a housewife, getting a meal is one link in an endless chain of household tasks. To a working woman, it may be a fine rest from an adding machine. The housewife would probably find it restful to run an adding machine a couple of hours a week. Learning to juggle stresses intelligently can become a very pleasant accomplishment.

Every woman, if she is to cope with the fatigue problem, needs not only planned rest and some time to herself, but also recreation and some way to express her creative talent. In my first book I wrote this advice to women: 'Stop being just a housewife.' One letter I got came from a husband who wanted desperately to help his wife do just that. She was getting dragged out by housework and care of their three-year-old, he said. He knew she had talents that were rusting away. Would I think it a good idea for him to encourage her to take a part-time job or do some volunteer work? I would, indeed. Even a routine type of activity that gets a woman out of the house a few hours a week will break the circle of monotony, give her something new to think about, put new zest into her life, make her feel more of a whole person.

I believe the lack of such outlets is the reason some mothers consider working or wish they could consider it. Taking care of a home and a baby does not fulfil a kind of inner yearning they have. There should be some way for such a mother to find the things that can augment her home life, help her make the kind of life she wants for herself. Perhaps it may be through the church, or the Home and School or Parent-Teacher Association, or other community affairs, that she can stretch her horizons and her life.

Years ago in my home town, Morrisburg, Ontario, my mother always had two great interests outside our home – the church and the Board of Education. But Mother had no problems of geography or transportation. We lived across from the church and it was a five-minute walk to the Board of Education office. She could encompass the whole thing almost within sight of home, and, as I remember, she did! A mother in a modern city can find all kinds of things to do, too, but it takes more planning – and more energy.

Every woman can and should find something to stimulate her mind and heart, if only because her home and family take on a new significance when she comes home with a new idea. The big questions are what, and how much to do? This is where an assessment is in order. There has to be enough to act as a stimulator but not so much that outside responsibilities worry her.

You have no idea how often a woman has a backache because of something that has very little to do with the condition of her spine! Sometimes she thinks her internal organs are out of place. When examination shows her back is fine and her insides in perfect order, I know I must find out more about her life – what she is doing, what time she gets up, when she takes her rest periods. Sometimes it takes a while to get to some clue to that backache. It may go something like this:

'Have you any children?'

'Yes, four.'

'They go to school?'

'Yes.'

'Do they come home to lunch?'

'One of them does. The others are away all day.'

(She shouldn't have a backache, I say to myself.)

'How many rooms are there in your house?'

'Six.'

'Any stairs?'

'Yes.'

'How many times a day do you go up and down stairs?'

'Oh, about every half-hour.'

'You go up and down stairs every half-hour! What for?'

'Well, I have my mother living with me and she's not very well.'

(Or, maybe, instead of her mother being confined to bed, it's that her father has a little trouble with his memory and she has to watch him as she would a child.)

Only then do I see that the reason for her backache is that she is just burdened, burdened by her old folks. And I know the next thing to do is to settle down and find a way to divide that burden or alleviate it in some other way.

In my country the old age pension, to which all our old folks are entitled at age seventy, brings extra income in such homes. This can be used for help with laundry, cleaning, or ironing. But more often than not the extra income has been 'set aside for something special'. This is when I move in on her. 'Put that money back into the current account,' I say sternly. 'Get some help in the house. Those special things can wait.'

'What are we going to do with the old folks?' This is a problem I hear a lot about from tired women struggling against odds to make a happy family life.

Sometimes an older woman or man is able to bring kindness, respect and real helpfulness to add to the family happiness.

But very often there is a problem. It may involve

small things like Grandfather's not approving of a fifteen-year-old boy who wants to go around in blue jeans. More often it's a big thing like the old person's requiring so much attention from mother that she isn't able to give her children the kind of attention they need. This simply can't be. A mother's first responsibility is always to her husband and her children.

It's one thing to have Grandfather and Grandmother come to visit for a certain length of time; deciding to make a home for the old folks is quite another. This decision should be made by looking at the whole situation and asking: is it possible or not? If it's made without thought or real planning, the mother winds up, like my patient, telling me or some other doctor, 'I have a backache.' What she's really saying is, 'I'm dead tired. How am I going to manage?'

I don't think one can make any set rules about what to do about young people or old people, or when you should have children, or when a wife should work. But I do think each big decision must be measured against the happiness of a home and a total family.

I do suggest that a couple should have six months to themselves before they begin their family. Sometimes this is hard to accept, especially by couples who have waited to marry until their early thirties. I think it's better for the future of the family that the husband and wife have at least six months to think only of each other before they learn to be father and mother, which necessarily means thinking of a third person in the family.

As a doctor I approve of women having babies when

young, and I'm also in favour of larger families, providing the babies aren't spaced so closely that it threatens the mother's health. I always add that women who have their families when they are young should think ahead and prepare themselves for another big span of life when their children will be grown and they will still be young and vigorous. They should get enough education so they will be able to fill this part of their life with interesting work of some kind.

Marriage is a way of life for two people in which each grows in grace, beauty and love of life. A happy marriage does not depend on having children nor on financial success. It depends on the ability of the partners to make a home which will be for all members of the family a place to be re-created. For a real home is a resting place on the journey of life. It doesn't make the journey easier, but it gives the strength to make the journey.

What makes a happy family? You might say it takes two people in perfect health, to begin with. Yet I have a patient who has had a serious heart condition for years, and has had two babies and made a beautiful family life. She must take good care of herself, of course; she gets up at ten o'clock, rests two hours in the afternoon, and must strictly limit her activities. But she has put so much of the love of God into her home that her family is one of the happiest in town. The whole family can revolve around sickness and take it.

Another of my patients is a deaf-mute and so is her husband. They have been trained to speak a little, but I can't understand them very well. Their six-year-old daughter acts as a kind of interpreter, so I have come to know her and feel what a happy little girl she is. Should they have had a child? Well, why not? They make a wonderful job of it. Should the heart patient who might live only six months or two years more have had her babies? Of course. Health is important and I don't minimize it, but it isn't the only thing, nor the most important ingredient in happy family living.

Love is what holds a family together. Anything that chokes off love or destroys it makes the family fall apart. Because I believe this so firmly, I have this way of thinking of a family – as an intimate little group which is making a kingdom of heaven. Not that we don't fall short of it, at best, and, at worst, make quite the opposite of it.

The small child learns simple things about what he sees – for instance, that he must not touch the stove that is glowing with heat. But he also learns about things that neither he nor we can see. He grows in the knowledge of love given – or not given.

You never know when your outgoing spirit, the certain knowledge of your love, a moment of insight into you as a person, will touch deep into the heart of your child and fasten there for ever.

A mother is a bulwark of her home. Keeping everything together, including herself, takes some doing. If her family is happy, it's well worth it; women always say so.

9

Too Tired to Love

A HAPPY BEDROOM takes on the attributes of a sanctuary to a married couple. Within these four walls, husband and wife reach the height and the depth of the expression of their life together. If they both feel that this is a resting place for them to keep returning to, their children will also feel it.

I remember, as a child, rushing home after school and shouting for mother, as every child does, then running upstairs to the big bedroom which was mother's and father's and finding mother sitting by the big window, sewing. She could have sewed downstairs in the living-room, or even in the kitchen, but no, she was sewing by the lovely bright window in the bedroom. We all came to feel that this room was a sanctuary to her, the place where she was most at ease in her home.

Every bedroom can be happy if a woman will learn where her happiness lies and that it comes about differently from the way her husband's does. This takes knowledge, search, patience, humour, and love. It is rare for a couple to achieve their dreams when they first marry.

What things detract from the happy bedroom? The first and most important is fatigue. No doubt about it, a happy sex life takes energy! When a woman is tired out, her emotional life is at a dead level. A sense of defeat and disillusionment follows when she begins to doubt her ability to love and make love.

Girls who are about to get married should understand this. Too often they are tired out from the beginning of their marriages, exhausted from the bridal showers, the shopping, the parties, and the many decisions which accompany this very important step in a girl's life. A tired bride does not make a happy and energetic partner in love.

A young patient of mine called me the morning after her wedding from her honeymoon retreat, three thousand miles away. Weeping inconsolably she said, 'Last night wasn't anything like I thought it would be. It was my fault. What will I do?'

'What happened?' I asked, already having a hunch. She had been tired when I'd seen her several weeks before. Since then the newspaper had reported parties in honour of her and her fiancé almost daily, ending with yesterday's huge church wedding.

'I love George. Really I do. But I couldn't seem to *feel* much of anything. I just wanted to go to sleep.'

'No wonder,' I said briskly. 'It's too bad you were so short on rest and sleep working up to your wedding that you had to fall apart when it was over. George is probably exhausted too. But cheer up, things will get better. Take it easy a couple of days and let nature take its course. In forty-eight hours you'll both be laughing about it.'

She hung up, after begging me not to tell anyone she had called. Of course I didn't. When she came home she came in to see me, and we both laughed about her moment of panic. Sure enough, George had been tired out too. When they had talked it over, she found he had been worried for fear the fiasco had been *his* fault; then they had done a sensible thing – blamed the whole thing on fatigue and forgotten about it.

I believe in short honeymoons. For all its joy, it is wearing on the nervous system to learn about love-making and all the other things that go with this new way of life with someone. The learning should be interspersed with things that are familiar, where one feels at home.

Later, if a girl is working and beginning to have a family, the demands on her energy multiply, and her fatigue deepens. Loving may become increasingly hard. Joy may seldom light up the sky.

Many a wife has a take-it-or-leave-it feeling about love-making. My own estimate is that at least half of the married women are not frightfully interested. Sometimes they really are unusually tired because of some worry or because of caring for growing children. Many younger women who are afraid of becoming pregnant because they don't want to give up their jobs or for some other reason will use fatigue as an excuse. Others, after ten or twelve years of marriage when the glamour has worn off, will develop symptoms to serve them in this way. I have had women bring me lengthy lists of symptoms, hoping they could go home and tell their husbands, 'The doctor says I can't.'

On the other hand, many women have come to me to find out how they can get their husbands interested in a sex life again. This happens more often than you would think. Women are ashamed to admit it.

One patient complained, 'Honestly, all he thinks of is his job and getting ahead. I want another baby so badly, but he seems indifferent.'

Having a baby had been a wearing experience for this couple. After several years of trying, they had come to me for help. When she finally did get pregnant, she had an uneasy time of it and a difficult delivery. The husband adored their little boy, but it was easy to understand that he might not want to go through such a trying time again very soon.

'Give him time,' I counselled. 'He had to go right on earning your living while you were having such a hard time getting the first baby. Work at keeping yourself in good shape and let him get his feet on the ground.'

Eventually she did get pregnant again, and this time the whole thing went more easily.

It is sad to me that women note that they feel indifferent to love-making and stop there. They need to understand that making love with their husbands is not just a physical phenomenon. It engages the mind and heart as well as the body. For her own sake as well as her husband's, she must work to create that atmosphere of love which is a communication of body, mind, and particularly heart, so that love-making becomes a renewing of the whole creature. A woman can do this both well and easily. And ecstasy can be part of it for her without her having to experience the same kind of physical excitement and fulfilment that her husband feels.

Both partners must realize this. I find it awfully difficult to make a husband understand that his wife's happiness in the art of making love is not necessarily of the same type or quality as his own.

Once they get over this hurdle, these two people who are so very different – male and female – begin to discover what they can achieve together. Then they can create such a happy relationship of body, mind, and spirit in the very depth of their love-making!

If all marriage partners could reach this understanding, all wives would be interested in a full sex life.

Sometimes I think married couples could achieve the happy bedroom more successfully in a tent than in a well-furnished flat where distracting things are apt to be going on. In my first book I emphasized this next point but, judging from letters I have received, men still do not realize that a woman's attention is easily distracted during the act of love. If someone just walks along the hall, she becomes wary. If the telephone rings, if a car stops in the street – all perfectly natural occurrences – it distracts her. That's her nature. She can't help it.

Fatigue overtakes not only the married woman who is unable to find success and happiness in her love life with her husband, but also the unmarried woman who has no husband with whom to make love. I am in a position to know that each envies the other! When night falls after a long day of seeing patients, I sometimes have a fanciful vision: all the married women are busily thinking up ways to avoid making love, and all the unmarried women are just dying to get at it!

It is a fact that in the menopause women usually lose interest in sex relations. Most married women would like to announce to their husbands that they are giving up their love life for a while!

But this is very unwise. Life goes on. And this indifference is temporary. Once a woman has passed the menopause, her interest in her sex life comes back, usually in all its glory and sometimes even more so.

A far more worrisome difficulty, as Professor Kinsey pointed out, is that when the husband comes to his period of decline, which is very like the menopause, his interest in sex life may continue to diminish, rather than reviving as the woman's interest does.

Whatever their fatigue and lack of interest, I urge women not to give up their sex lives during menopause. In the first place, this is a transient period. In the second place, a woman must hold together this important part of her marriage. No matter that it is not exciting to her. A continuing sex life is necessary to her as well as to her husband, for the simple reason that it preserves and nourishes the marriage at a time when she needs the security of that marriage.

When a mother comes for her final examination after she has had her baby, we talk about her resuming her sex life with her husband. Something new is going to develop in their physical relationship, I explain to her. As they go back and pick up this part of their life together, they will feel a great tenderness which can keep growing in them throughout their life together.

But often the patient will say, 'We are just too tired to start yet.'

'You may be too tired,' I say to her, 'but I doubt that your husband is. Your love together is just as important now as it ever was, and you must take care of it. You feed your child so it will grow in stature. Just so, it's up to you and your husband to nurture your marriage and see that the child grows up in a happy home.'

In most marriages at some time, a wife or husband will withhold their love life from each other because they are distracted, hurt, or excited. This is a powerful weapon because it is the one that hurts the worst. It is a temptation to use it when a person feels personally wounded. But it is one of the things a marriage partner should never do. It is a sin against the spirit.

Another thing that often creeps in to destroy the love life of a couple is just plain boredom. A woman or man, particularly a woman, can be really hurt by the partner's being a dull, bored lover. A happy married life does not grow from doing the same thing in the same way at the same time. Feeling and fun must be kept alive. Both partners must keep pouring out their life and love to keep their marriage growing.

Separation presents a different but definite problem. Some men have to be away because of business except for the week-end; others must go regularly for a longer time. Every possible means should be employed by both husband and wife to keep the husband as intimately connected with his home while he is away as when he is there. In the times they are together they can renew their feeling, revitalize their love for each other. Gradually they can grow into a new relationship.

We get out of life exactly what we put into it. So it is with the cultivation and nurture of love.

The extra effort that makes a marriage worth while is sometimes buried under the burden of household routine or feelings of disappointment and resentment which a woman may allow to accumulate. She plays her hand masterfully in snaring a man, but drops the strategy after marriage. I believe this to be one of the greatest weaknesses of marriage.

A favourite patient and also a great friend of mine was one of those women who, instead of showing the depth of nervous and emotional tension in headaches, backaches, or stomach spasms, had profuse periods. At three critical times in her life these became so severe she could not work. She had had a run of extraordinarily bad luck following the loss of her husband by a tragic, sudden death, when her two children were babies. Then she had been engaged after a time, but the plans were broken by mutual consent but with sorrow on both sides. After an interval she came into my office, engaged again and completely transformed. I examined her and sent her on her way, delighted that she had found happiness and a home at last.

A year later she was on my schedule again. She was

haemorrhaging, her blood count was down and her spirits even lower. There was a blank, life-isn't-fair look in her eyes.

Every person who enters marriage comes to the point when at last she sees her mate for exactly what he is. In the first months or years of being truly in love, no one can hear or see the truth of the beloved. And thank God for that!

'He doesn't pay his bills,' my patient's inventory of injury began, 'and he drinks a little too much. He's had two jobs in a year. I'm afraid to quit mine because we need the money. At night I come home to get dinner and he stops for a drink with the boys.' To top it all off, her children by her previous marriage were becoming problems. Her new husband refused to discipline them himself, and took sides with the children when she tried to do it.

Tough as it is, this situation has been faced by thousands of women before. The expectation that a man will support them and make a home for them cannot be realized. They hoped to be protected, but find that they must be the strong ones. This is a time to count up one's assets and realize that one's love and desire to make a marriage work are meeting a supreme test.

When we had discussed this a little, she said, 'But I don't respect him any more. How can I respond to his love-making when I feel the way I do?'

'Wait a minite,' I said. 'That's the silliest statement of all. Your respect for him when you married him was not based on any record of his achievements. You knew that he was a risk. You can't sit in judgement on him now. First of all, you have to accept him for what he is – a lovable, happy-go-lucky companion. You like his charm, his good looks, the way he makes you laugh. But he's forty years old and you can't start remoulding him now. Just a little while ago he would light up your eyes and your heart and your whole life – and he can still do that if you'll only shut your eyes to things he can't do: grow up and be masterful, take on the responsibility of a wife, a ready-made family, and his own affairs.'

When she had been so ecstatically in love, she couldn't see the truth about her husband. Now that life was real, she couldn't feel the ecstasy. But, I told her, 'You can know the finest love of all – compassion. You may ask me how you can respond to his love-making, but I say you can go farther than that. You can woo and comfort his distress, for he knows his limitations and he loves you.'

'This is all very well, but I have to work all day and then come home and get dinner while he stops to have a drink with his friends. It's not fair.'

'Of course it's not fair,' I agreed fervently. 'It never has and never will be fair. Let's forget about everything but you. First I want you to be well, so that you have your gay vitality of last year back again. Rest your worries and rest your weary body too. When you come from work, get some nourishment, put your feet up, let the drive of the day gradually slip away while you find out what happened at school today. Your children will love to find you listening again. As soon as this resting place is happier and more peaceful than some nearby bar, your husband will come home quickly too. The evening chores can be done all together, and you can be enthroned on the couch like a queen, beautiful as ever, by 9 p.m.'

As a doctor, I knew I must insist on the rest. As her friend, I felt she was worn out with thinking and judging, that she should be still for a while and let love catch her up again. She would find that a love full of compassion and giving would be a more wonderful, truer love because it would be built on real knowledge of her husband and no false expectations.

She had been expecting her husband to love her because she had been a good wife. It doesn't work that way. A woman loves her husband and children without stint or protection and, in so doing, inevitably makes her home a true resting place. Though there are hard days, she will have made it possible for her family to walk a little straighter, to know a small victory. They will not be afraid of life, for they will have the certain knowledge that they belong together.

Human beings can fail, but love can't and will find the way.

10

Shadows Cast by Our Modern Way of Life

WE THINK of great social changes as occurring in other parts of the world – India, Africa, China. So they do. But just as great changes take place right here at home.

My generation came from families in which the patterns of living were pretty well laid down and fairly rigid. But there was a stability about it. I look back on childhood and girlhood as a wonderful, glorious experience of life. It was a kind of free period before going into another quite rigid pattern. (From what we saw of our friends and relatives we could see that getting married imposed restrictions.)

Today the family pattern isn't rigid at all. In the first place, families live and move on wheels. The minute school is out, the whole family takes off. In the second place, the drudgery is gone. What with appliances and cake mixes coming in the door, drudgery has flown out of the window. Time was when a girl getting married was in a twit learning to cook. Today she just has to know how to open a frozen food package.

Today young women have free access to education. My mother had to insist that her daughters have the same chance for an education as her sons. Now everyone accepts the fact that any girl who has the ability can have the kind of education she can absorb.

Today money is easier to come by. Even boys and girls can earn substantial amounts if they want to work week-ends and summers. But at the same time the cost of living soars.

I have noticed that often a boy and girl feel they are making enough to get married because they can support each other, but they look at their earnings and overlook the cost of living, simply because up to this point the money they wanted has been easy to get.

I saw a girl who was being married a week before graduation from university. 'Don't you think you could wait another fifteen minutes?' I asked her. It did seem as if she was kind of missing something! Later in the conversation I found that both she and her fiancé were going on to graduate school. 'Forgive me for being blunt,' I said, 'but who is going to buy the bacon?' I was astonished to see that the high cost of living had not entered into their plans.

Along with early marriages (in fact, maybe even 'early' isn't quite the word for it) girls are planning to have more children. 'I was brought up where there were just two of us, or one of us, and I am going to have lots of children,' some of them say. Others seem to have slightly bizarre reasons.

A patient came to me recently and said, 'I would like to have another child.'

'Take it easy,' I said. 'I'd like you to wait a while.'

'But, Doctor,' she wailed, 'all my friends are having their third.'

'Never mind about that,' I said. 'Two will be enough for you for quite a while.'

'But' – she really believed this clinched her case – 'I can't let them get ahead of me.'

This kind of thing puzzles me. This woman, like the many others who have somewhat the same kind of attitude, is an intelligent person. I sense in them the feeling that they must find something important enough to give energy and real thought to. Having more children solves the problem for them. I am all for families, naturally, but I am for women taking their place in the world too. Sometimes I'm tempted to think they are trying to escape from doing so.

The fact that women work is something we have gotten used to. But today in the United States (and Canadian figures are running nearly as high) one third of all women in the country work, thirty per cent of all married women work, and nearly two out of five mothers whose children are school age are in the labour force. Women over age forty-five make up thirty-seven per cent of the female labour force, a rate which was predicted for 1970. What the National Manpower Council refers to as 'a revolution in women's employment' has happened so fast it's unbelievable, but it's fact.

Young people are marrying earlier and having larger families ... Family life is altering in structure, patterns of family living becoming more fluid ... Women have free access to education ... Money flows more freely ...

Both the cost of living and the standard of living are rising ... More and more women are working, particularly married women, women with children, and women past forty-five.

Change is always interesting, and these changes are all very much so. On the face of it, one might merely be impressed with how dynamic they all sound. They're dynamic, all right. There's so much going on in modern civilization that has to do with women's lives and their roles, biological and social, that most of us feel we have to keep a stiff upper lip and a cool head to avoid being overwhelmed completely.

Yet, as a woman and a women's doctor, I feel that women have only begun to find themselves and to realize their potentialities.

Our modern way of life lightens women's lives; at the same time it casts shadows over their lives. Women have handier kitchens, supermarkets, permanent waves, electrically-run gadgets to bear the brunt of many household chores, and these are all to the good.

I can think of many shadows cast by our modern way of life, but I want to discuss four which I think are particularly disturbing to women's happiness and well-being: the drive of modern life, our shifting values, loneliness, and a pervasive confusion between love and passion.

What a circus act we women perform in the life of multiplicity we lead! We drive ourselves – to look after a home, to do a job, to keep up with the neighbours, to win – or keep – the reputation as the smartest hostess or best clubwoman in town. Not only are legitimate deadlines imposed on us, but we make others for ourselves in order to accomplish so much in a given time.

This drive of modern civilization is felt not only by working women. Everyone will recognize these familiar faces: The woman who makes a full-time job of competing with her neighbours and best friends. The young executive's wife who is expected by the company to compete with wives of executives of rival companies. The mother of three eligible daughters. The woman who is not content with keeping up with the Joneses but must pass them *en route*.

Such a drive bores into life, hits directly into the control of the nervous system, and may pass into the hormonal structure so that a woman enters the stage of fatigue where she can no longer adapt herself.

Here's a sporting proposition. Stop right now and take stock of all the things that are driving you. How much of it is accumulated from sheer momentum because you've driven yourself past a certain point and can't stop?

Modern women have to find a quiet time of the day for themselves, a time for letting the drive of life disappear. Some women have so many demands on them from so many directions that they can't find five minutes that is their own unless they work at planning for it.

One of the lovely things about doing obstetrics is you seldom have a problem of conflicting demands. When the mother is going to have her baby, you go with her. Patients may have to sit and wait in the office. The family may have to go on with the dinner-party without you. Somebody else may have to be pressed into service to make the speech at the reunion dinner. You sit quietly and wait with the mother to have the baby. Even when you do it around the clock, there is still no problem about the drive of life. You know what you have to do. Your priority is set for you.

It is the noise of modern life that destroys the soul. If a woman neglects her own personal security, then when the noise stops there is no inner music.

My friend Sue gets up a half-hour earlier than she used to, just so she can organize her day in peace and quiet. Most of my patients who work find the best quiet time is when they get home from their jobs. They can put their feet up and rest until the 'push' is gone.

You may say, 'But I must get dinner.' The fact is that eating, like sleeping, is an adjustable sort of thing. When I come home at half past seven or quarter of eight, the housekeeper always wants to rush dinner to the table. 'The poor girl,' she thinks, 'she must be starved.' What I really want is to sit down for a half-hour's peace before I eat.

Much has been said and written about the shift in our culture towards materialistic values. I do not know why, when we have the whole history of human experience to teach us, we should have allowed it to happen. Could it be that, as it did with my friend and patient, Amy, it kind of crept up on civilization?

Amy is married to a businessman and has a fine family of four youngsters, ranging from sixteen-year-old Tom down to ten-year-old Patty. Amy is an expert statistician and has worked for years, with time out for maternity leaves, for a firm in a Canadian city. She loves her family – and her job – and is fortunate enough to have had the same part-time housekeeper, a widow with grown children, for nearly fifteen years.

Five years ago Amy came to me on the point of exhaustion. Her fatigue was peculiar to the women who suffer from this thing I call 'the drive of modern life'. Their problem arises from an all-out effort to possess the best of two worlds – family life and job life, an effort which too often wins them the worst of both.

These women rise early, do part of their work at home, get to their place of business on time. During the day they can relax briefly, if they are lucky. If they hold jobs of great importance, they may not have a real break all day. At day's end they speed through rush-hour traffic, supervise the dinner hour and evening chores (some do it all themselves). The work they do on the job is considerable. Added to their home responsibilities, it builds up a drive that keeps a woman's metabolism in a state of bombardment.

To get back to Amy, she was a mess – too tired to enjoy her lively family and so under par that she could scarcely make sense out of the requests for computations that came to her office desk. Having to get up at six-thirty had begun to assume nightmare proportions. Dinner-table conversation, usually a sprightly interlude in their family life, had fallen off. Her husband retired gloomily behind his paper each evening. The housekeeper had given up trying to please Amy and was dropping hints about leaving.

It took some doing to rouse a spark of interest on Amy's part in the problem that had rolled up. She had come with the vague idea that I could give her pills or a booster shot of some kind. Finally we got her schedule laid out, piece by piece. I found that she had taken on extra work at the office, which meant that she ate lunch at her desk several times a week. Knowing that in the past she had enjoyed meeting friends for lunch, I realized she had cut down on a daily period of relaxation. Why had she taken on the extra work? For the extra money, she said – it would swell the fund for the children's education. Also, she added hurriedly, it might lead to a promotion.

The older children were then moving into a phase of taking lessons in this and that, joining clubs, bringing their friends home. Amy was spending Saturdays chauffeuring them hither and yon, frenziedly trying to keep up her reputation as brilliant party-giver, good mother, cook *par excellence* – and working overtime at the office.

'Stop it,' I told her. 'Slow down to a walk. You don't really need that extra money. What good is it to the children if their mother is an invalid? Besides, they can earn part of their own education. As for a promotion, you're in no shape now to accept one. Get yourself back in focus. If you feel badly about your family life, try putting more into it and putting it first.'

I am happy to report that Amy overhauled her home-job priority list promptly. In a surprisingly short time she had herself and her family back on an even keel.

I am all for women working. But women with dual responsibilities of work and home must go in for thorough assessment of themselves and the stress their obligations will put upon them. They must decide how they are going to make life happy for themselves and their families.

For some mothers who work full time and under pressure and do their own work at home, it may be wiser to lengthen the waking hours than to go at a rapid pace. It seems a very hard thing but, even if they already get up at six-thirty, it really is better to shift to a six o'clock rising hour. If they work more slowly during the morning, and rest a little when they come home from their jobs in the afternoon, they are better able to take on the next job. A woman like Amy should take a half-hour to let the drive of the job seep out of her system before she starts dinner. By such a simple adjustment the change of pace from the wear and tear of business life to house-keeping tasks can become beneficial. Many working women have learned to make it a refreshing avocation.

A great many married women have to work to earn a living or to add to family resources. Women with husbands who are disabled, unskilled, or who perhaps don't pay the bills. Widows with families. Women whose husbands have suffered some great financial upset or job loss.

When should a woman *choose* to work? Not because she has to but because she would like to.

A married woman who wants to go to work must first look at the 'Why?' in her own reasoning. Is she running from something? Is it that she just can't stand doing house-work any longer? Has she had too much of caring for little children? Is it because she is nervous and wants to get her mind off herself?

I believe all work is of equal value. The kind of work you do isn't so important as what you feel about that kind of work. A woman can do a wonderful job at keeping her house clean and feel fine about it, or she can feel like a menial. Nurses and doctors can hate the difficult, smelly chores that go with their jobs, or they can accept them as part of a total job they love doing.

Nevertheless I have been astonished to see how much happier some married women have been when they return to work. In doing even small jobs which require no training, they feel more valued by the community than they were as housewives. The truth is that married women who keep house and care for a family of three or four children are not only hard workers but extremely valuable ones. Their jobs are constant, continuous, going round the clock. The product of their labours is our most important national asset – the next generation of men and women. But it is difficult for many women to win the feeling of achievement which they so well deserve. Our gadget-ridden society has cut them off from some of the really satisfying work in a home, and husbands aren't as appreciative as they might be.

The tired businessman coming home to the overwrought wife, while it is such an old story it is a cliché situation, is still not one conducive to mutual appreciation.

'Not only does he come home tired,' said a weary wife in my office recently, 'but he's so busy trying to be a man in a grey flannel suit, he can't relax and be himself even then.'

'And what are you trying to be?' I asked.

She thought a moment.

'Decorative, I guess,' she said. 'But I can't even get up to the level of a Class B movie star.'

How many people are goaded by modern advertising to be something other than what they are, to be someone else! Life is real. Struggling to approximate the human symbols of our mass media is quite a trick at any age; after thirty-five or forty, it's a losing battle.

If a woman chooses to work, she must fulfil that very basic need of any person – the need for a sense of achievement. Therefore she must work for some good reason, not just to get the money for a refrigerator, the down payment on a house, or just to get the money, period. She must work because she gets that wonderful sense of giving, contributing, creating. If her work calls for little imagination and creative ability, it can still give her a feeling of achievement, of being an asset to the world.

I am convinced that the loneliness which is peculiar to our modern way of life, and which, curiously enough, results from our efforts to increase comfort and bring about better living conditions, is a cause of fatigue.

The development of suburbia is the example that comes most readily to mind. It has been interesting to me to see the women who have moved, sometimes when they were scarcely able to afford it, to a new suburb. They looked forward to it with great pleasure. They like having plenty of room for the children. They feel the whole family will take a new lease on life. Then gradually they find they have fewer and fewer friends and little communication with people outside their immediate families. Often they are confined to their homes because of their small children. If this is a one-car family, the wife is marooned after the man of the house wheels off to work in the morning.

A kind of fatigue grows up out of sheer loneliness. It is not that these women are bored, for they are busy and get enjoyment from having the home they have always dreamed of. Loneliness is a better word for it.

Old people living by themselves, young people moving away from the family into their own establishments. All have loneliness to cope with. Many suffer from fatigue. I do not say that these modern developments are not very good. But in gaining the comfort and convenience of having one's own place, or taking the children to better surroundings, one loses some of the comforts of the spirit.

We cannot survive without communication with others. Day by day a kind of fatigue and tiredness seep into the soul of the person who is cut off from companionship. It is one of the most devastating things that can happen. When the whole of life is lived essentially alone, the way is opened to fears of all sorts. The contact of one individual with another, even though it may be fraught with difficulties, is better than not having any. Social studies have proved this. Most of us have learned it from our own experience.

The person who wants to communicate with others but finds it difficult to do so because of factors within himself, rather than because of geographical distances, suffers from the most desolate, defeated feelings a person can have. One must have affection. As the body takes food for its nutrition, so the intellectual and emotional life of the person is nourished by ideas, opinions, feelings, and experiences shared with others. A doctor is aware of the nearness of complete breakdown by the way a person withdraws. Because the person is so frightfully insecure, he cannot risk the interplay of human emotions, and his health diminishes.

Loneliness is such a penetrating emotion that I think of it first. But fatigue follows in the wake of every bitter emotion known to the human race and prolongs them all, for the sufferer from these emotions becomes too tired to cure herself.

Our modern way of life has plucked a great group of young adult women from the midst of family, school, and community and set them down again in large cities. Here they earn a living in an office, a factory, a store, or in some professional capacity. Here they live in a room, a small bachelor apartment, or share an apartment with other girls. Some marry and build a home and family. Some build a career. Some do both. Some just survive.

Trying to put down her own roots and make a life for herself is a struggle for this modern young woman.

A girl in her early thirties consulted me because she was having menstrual difficulties. A well-educated person, she had a good job which involved travelling part of the time, so she lived in a modest room in the city. She loved her job, but admitted her room seemed cramped and lonely, especially on week-ends.

When I had examined her and talked with her long enough to get a good picture of her life, I advised her to find an apartment.

'Your trouble comes from being tired of not having enough outside your job. You need a home of your own,' I said. 'If you have a friend who will take an apartment with you, so much the better. You can begin collecting furniture and pictures that you'll like living with, and entertaining your friends. You are too young and attractive and interesting to be as lonely as you are.'

Another patient, a professional woman in her late thirties, got into the bad habit of always being 'too tired to do anything'. It took time for her to realize she had gotten into a vicious circle: failure to offset the demands of the job with some social life had increased her fatigue and made her restless and cynically disinterested in everything, to boot.

'It's like homesickness,' she told me, when she was able to admit her loneliness. 'You know there's nothing really wrong with you, but there might as well be, you feel so bad.'

The tough time is in the thirties and early forties, when a woman finally knows the chances are she will not marry and have a family. It's not the end of the world;

it just seems like it. My prescription – and this has worked for hundreds of women – is to get enough rest, try to see yourself in perspective, work at getting an attitude of looking ahead and wondering what will come next, but most of all, absorb yourself in something interesting, preferably something you share with other people.

Three great problems confront these modern young women. The first is economic: they must keep a job and hope to advance. The second is sexual: they must learn to deal wisely with their female drives and desires. The third is a problem they have in common with the whole human race: they must find achievement and happiness as persons.

A single girl lets herself in for fatigue by playing outside her own league, as it were. It would be commonly accepted, I believe, that a girl in university shouldn't go about with a man who is thirty-five, divorced, knowledgeable about women; she is entirely outside the command of her own position. Just so, a secretary should never go out with her boss, if he is married or much older than she. Whether the man is unscrupulous or not, it isn't a wise thing to do. It is too easy for her to fall in love. Then, nature being what it is, this will become an affair in which two people are involved beyond their reason or ability to control it. It shouldn't get to the point where people are condemning a man for being unscrupulous. A girl must accept from the start that this kind of situation just doesn't work, and be content to stay in her own league.

I have often been asked if I 'believed' in platonic friendships. A friendship is only platonic when the man and woman together have faced the fact that they cannot become involved as lovers and set limits on themselves. If such a relationship is achieved, it will be because the man and woman have agreed to abide by the rule of conduct which they have laid down.

Letters I have had from women of Canada and the United States have disturbed and amazed me. 'Why must I spend my life without a man?' 'Tell the married women to stay with their own men and give us single women a chance.' 'It's very hard for a single woman to make her way because it's easier for a man to take out a married woman because it is so safe.' 'There must be another woman in the life of a successful man.' 'I am twenty-five. Life is over for me. I have no desire.'

What amazes me in these remarks is how ignorant women can be. They are misinformed about the obvious needs of a woman – of any human being – the need for status, achievement and affection. We are born with desire, but satisfaction of passion in mating is not among our truly basic needs. The need for love – genuine affection – *is* basic.

Confusion of love and passion is a very widespread cultural characteristic of our times. Why do we get the two mixed up? I think it comes from the fact that the power to love and the power of desire are both present in the infant. The feeling of physical desire becomes overlaid with spiritual warmth and understanding gradually, as the child grows up. Yet there can be a sudden empathy of minds and communication of spirit which shortly may overflow into a physical sense of nearness and closeness and a desire to express this spiritual communication by a communication of body. This feeling is natural to all men and women and can work in all directions. As there is no clear dividing line, we often become confused and mistake passion for love—or love for passion.

We must take care that our actions are constructive and nourishing to the whole personality, both our own and others'. This means behaving in a manner that doesn't cause destruction of ourselves or anyone else in the society in which we live.

Certain situations make for the sudden recognition and communication of two minds and hearts. Similarly, certain situations make for the sudden recognition and communication of two passionate desires. I want to stress particularly that one person can never know the depth of need another may have. Such a need may exert a strong pull, a positive drawing power. We all have to be mindful of other people as we go about our daily business, and be prepared to act as our brothers' keepers, if need be. This is particularly true when we come to physical desire.

I remember one patient who came rushing into my office one day and said, 'May I sit in your waiting-room for a while?'

'Of course, but why?' I asked.

'My husband brought home one of his business friends for dinner last night and something extraordinary happened to me. I was terribly attracted to this man. I almost felt I could melt into his arms if he held them out. I am a very happily married woman. I know, logically, that I don't want that man. I don't even want to see him again. If I can stay in your office during the day for a while, I'm sure I can work this out and it will pass.'

It is natural for every one of us to experience unaccountable attractions for other people. Sometimes, with the right timing and staging, these feelings can be almost violent. But they just cannot be allowed to develop because they may destroy ourselves or other people whom we care about. Sometimes women feel it is right to follow the command of these sudden desires because of the great need of the other person. Many a woman has entered into an affair because the feeling of being needed was so compelling. If her action contributes to the destruction of her own self-respect or the unhappiness of any other person, it is wrong.

Let us try now to put down in simple terms the difference between love and passion.

Passion is relentless, rushing into any vacuum, driving on to its own self-satisfaction regardless of the circumstances or the havoc which may follow. Passion has no morals, no standards, no control, and no compassion. It is cruel and devouring, looking only for its own immediate fulfilment. Passion tosses aside the rules, Christian ethics, civilization and individual plans and intentions. Passion disregards dignity and grace. It is humourless, full of rage.

Love, on the other hand, is more powerful than passion. Love illuminates all aspects of our relations between men and women, parents and child, friends and, ideally, between nations. Sometimes in the recognition of one spirit by another there is a sudden spark kindling an inspiration which may last a lifetime. Love never destroys. It is trusting like a child, tender like a lover, and tough like a mother. Love knows no social barriers, no age limits. For me, love implies the ability to accept the person just as she is. Love understands, respects, and is always willing to wait. Love listens, and love then gives. Love is also joyful and, at times, exquisitely and quietly humorous. Love can occur in many different guises, but when love between a man and a woman overflows into passion, the relationship is restored and recreated again and again. The marriage is then truly blessed.

But passion without love is disaster, and love without passion is no marriage. Love with passion but without the knowledge of how love is nurtured may wither, and vacuums may form. Time, imagination, laughter, and the rest are the prescriptions I give. Surely one of the best of all sounds that must come to the ears of God is the happy, tender, affectionate, understanding laughter of a husband and wife in the prelude of their love-making.

11

The Fallacy of the Short Cut to Vitality

WE WORRY about feeling tired. Our grandparents probably felt tired in their day, but no doubt took it for granted and didn't fret about it.

I think we worry because we have so much greater expectations of ourselves than they did. We must be successful. All successful people are brisk, bright, vital, and energetic – any advertisement will tell you so. In our culture fatigue is something one can't afford.

Yet we have it. And because of this dilemma, we glance at fatigue out of the corner of one eye, instead of looking it full in the face. We give it a disinterested nod, when we should get acquainted with it. Instead of treating it with the respect any real problem deserves, we take short cuts to get rid of it – a quick drink, a sleeping pill, Benzedrine.

Many people make a fetish out of short cuts. Many others make a lot of money out of them.

My new car will go slowly without stalling, fast without knocking – so fast I could pick up a traffic ticket almost without knowing it. It can be steered with the tip of a finger, stopped with the tip of the toe. It is warm when it's cold outside, and relatively cool when it's hot outside. At night its lights make the road almost as bright as day.

This is what we expect from our machines in modern society, and we often thoughtlessly expect the same of ourselves. We should wake up in the morning feeling fresh as a daisy, straining to get at the day's work. Midmorning and even mid-afternoon should find us still riding the crest of tremendous energy.

If we are to be interviewed by the boss we should be calm and imaginative. If we are interviewing one of our staff we should be clear and unemotional.

We should be hungry for our meals, yet not want to eat too much. After dinner at night we should feel as alert as we did in the morning, able to go on working or taking part in brilliant repartee. Sleep should come easily and be deep and restful.

That's what we sometimes expect our day to be like. Human flesh and the nervous system, however, were not made to run so perfectly in a world of fairly intimate human relationships full of stressful and frustrating situations.

A great many people feel they do not wake up completely rested. Many of us have some days at least when we can't seem to get started. Sometimes we try to remedy the lack of energy by some artificial means—extra coffee extra-strong, or some energizer or stimulant. If the stimulant is really helpful, we come to rely on it more and more frequently.

By mid-morning many people pause to catch their breath and have more coffee (or more Benzedrine). The real purpose of the coffee break is to interrupt the tempo of the morning and allow us a few minutes to relax and be sociable. The coffee is incidental; if we drink it, it should be because we like it, not merely because we think it's a safe stimulant.

Never a day goes by in a doctor's office that one or more patients do not complain of feeling tense. The next question is never 'What shall I do?' but invariably, 'Doctor, what shall I take?' Often the patient frankly admits knowing full well what she should do, but says she doesn't want to do it. Instead, she wants something to take.

Today we have a great variety of drugs available for waking up the human nervous system, stimulating it, soothing it, or putting it to sleep. While they are valuable to the doctor in treating sick people, their use has spread far beyond the boundaries of the sickroom.

These drugs are powerful chiefly because of the tremendous faith placed in them. They are harmful because they support the mistaken idea that the human animal should always be at ease, or always be at his or her best. Their continued use can be as fruitless as anything else that treats the result rather than the cause of a disorder. This is one of the oldest of medical problems; it has taken on a new look only because of the widespread use of the new drugs coming on to the market.

It is perfectly normal to be nervous when you go in to see the boss. Most people are. In fact, most bosses expect it. The impression you make when nervous is much better than when sedated with a tranquillizer or inspired by a stimulant.

The plain truth is that any short cut to overcoming our reticence, controlling our nervousness, or stimulating our confidence is harmful simply because it's artificial. When its effect wears off, a person is left with a sense of failure rather than a feeling of accomplishment.

Moreover, it postpones learning the normal techniques human beings can develop to gain much better results. Learning the technique of controlling nervousness, for instance, helps us use the nervousness for better performance. When we are nervous we can run faster, jump higher, think more quickly, and remember better. Some people get too fascinated with such unpleasant physiological evidences of nervousness as palpitations, sweating, and so on, and become frightened by them. It's better to look at nervousness as a pulling together of our energies – which it really is, or can be. Then we can have more confidence in what we are going to do *because* we are nervous, and the nervousness becomes a powerful aid in our effort to do our best.

If you have ever had the experience of making a speech when you were *not* nervous, you know it's just as easy to make a colossal failure of the whole thing under these circumstances as it is when your nervousness goes out of control.

Learning these techniques, such as controlling nervousness and overcoming shyness, is part of the job of learning to live satisfactorily. These are some of the things parents are called upon to help their children with. You can't teach it unless you've experienced it. Let us not limit what we can pass on to our children to the knowledge of when and how to use tranquillizers and stimulants.

In our modern life, with its demands and drives, alcohol is being used both as stimulant and tranquillizer. If you want to be the life of the party you are going to, you feel a cocktail enhances the chances. If you come home tired and want to relax, you take a cocktail to help you let down. You may feel alcohol helps you view a failure with complacency, or a challenge with confidence.

Alcohol is not universally successful on all these counts. For some people it may prove more relaxing than inspiring, so that they drowse through a party instead of sparkling through it, trying desperately to keep their eyes open. Actually, alcohol is not a stimulant, it's a depressant. One of the things it depresses is your critical faculties, so that you don't have the normal amount of inhibition. In some circles inhibition is frowned on as evidence of immaturity, and adults at a party are expected to be as gay and giddy as children. But whatever social circle you move in, you don't like to look back on a party evening and feel you've monopolized the conversation at length and in high key, or realize that the joke you thought screamingly funny at the time only succeeded in embarrassing someone else.

A colleague of mine from a foreign country once said to me, 'We wouldn't mind you Canadians and Americans working so hard and such long hours if you didn't make a virtue out of it.' It made me stop and think. In a curious sort of way, we do tend to make a virtue out of our excesses. For example, chain-smoking is often supposed to go along with the picture of the intent, creative, successful newspaper writer, advertising executive, or other glamourized figure in our civilization. By now anyone knows that excessive smoking affects a person's wind and circulatory system and produces in some people such bothersome and unpleasant symptoms as chronic coughs, hoarseness, and nausea on waking in the morning. But, like thumb-sucking, chain-smoking can only be cured by learning to feel at ease and confident of oneself. This seems to be hard for so many people in our society. It's easier to make a virtue out of the excess.

People know when they are smoking or drinking too much, but they keep on asking doctors if *they* think so, and if they do, do they think it's dangerous? Any excess is serious if it contributes to the deterioration of the spiritual self and one's nervous and physical functions.

Fatigue, as well as boredom and unhappiness, is temporarily relieved by drinking; if a person continues to drink to excess, fatigue ultimately becomes a chronic state. There is some debate among doctors as to whether alcohol is a poison or whether it is harmful merely because it is used to replace nourishing food. One reason this has been difficult to prove one way or the other is that different nervous systems respond differently to alcohol. There are people who for years have drunk too much, yet they continue to perform creditably in the office, on the stage, or over the air.

I believe these are exceptions. The nervous system of the average person cannot remain healthy if the person drinks excessively. Eventually he will begin to suffer from the shaky hand, failing vision, and faltering memory, even when he is entirely free of alcohol. One of the sad truths about that very vital part of our anatomy, the nervous system, is that it is easily damaged, the important parts being damaged first. Repair is possible, but often must be incomplete. A doctor is saddened at such a development just as a painter would be by the wilful spoiling of an exquisitely executed canvas, or a musician by the careless destruction of a fine instrument.

In most alcoholics I have tried to help, I saw beneath the pitiable, uncertain, bewildered exterior traces of a lovable, sensitive person who tried to do something beyond his or her capacity or kept making an effort against too discouraging odds. One girl I knew, a pianist, did awfully well in popular and semi-classical playing for variety programmes, but the effort to succeed in concert work was too much for her. She began to drink and her career went downhill. If she had not stopped drinking altogether, she would have lost out even in the field where she could succeed.

When alcohol can spell trouble for a woman is when she is demanding more of herself than she should have to, especially without the support of an understanding husband or friends, in a social environment which normally includes cocktails before dinner and after-dinner drinking. I have had many patients who expected themselves to be the perfect hostess to their husbands' business associates, including those who landed suddenly in town at the end of a day when these mothers were tired from caring for small children and making the round of household chores. Some of these patients have crossed the line between the relaxing pick-me-up and the 'drink I have to have to get me through the evening' without knowing it. There is a world of difference between a pleasant social custom and a crutch that seems to provide needed support.

Entertaining her husband's business friends grew to be a way of life for a long-time patient of mine. Because of her husband's business ventures, her home became a drop-in centre for assorted groups of people from the advertising, publicity, radio, and television worlds. Having writers and actors around, holding story conferences at odd hours of the day and night made an interesting, stimulating life for her, but made it impossible to maintain a normal ménage for herself, her husband, and their teen-age daughter. She began to drink too much just to stay in the swim. Each time I saw her she was more nervous and more tired.

I tried to help stem the tide and make her aware that she was headed for trouble. I couldn't get to first base. It was 'necessary for business reasons'. But life catches up with people in unexpected ways. One day when she came into my office I saw at once the snowballing had come to an end.

'Betty's getting married,' she said, lighting a cigarette

with a shaking hand. 'Just like that. No warning at all. He's a nice enough boy, but he's so – so pedestrian. A time-clock puncher in somebody's office.'

'Is it really that upsetting?' I asked.

She began to cry.

'No,' she admitted, between sobs. 'It's what she said, when we asked her to wait a while.'

'And what was that?'

'That – that she couldn't wait to get away from home.'

'Did she say why?' Mentally I was cheering Betty on.

'Yes,' she said in bewilderment, 'because she wants to have a home of her own where she can have meals at the same time every day. Imagine! Sure we live kind of a hectic life, but Betty's had everything a girl could want – everything!'

'Not quite everything, I'm afraid,' I commented carefully.

Betty's rejection of her parents' way of life got them down to brass tacks after they recovered from the first shock and put some thought on it. They faced the fact that excessive drinking was making inroads on them both and decided they had been looking at things the wrong way around. They did not have to drink for business reasons; in fact, if they had to live a fast-paced, irregular life because of business, they'd better not drink at all. They went on the wagon together. This was important, I thought. The support they could give each other was extremely helpful to both.

This couple found the world didn't come to an end

when they began carrying around glasses of unspiked ginger ale at parties. Far from it. They began to look better, feel better, enjoy both business and social life more.

'And,' said my patient, 'I feel like a human being in the morning!'

Drinking to escape uncertainty, worry and unhappiness, and unpleasant home life is senseless but all too common.

Another patient kept herself going on alcohol through her husband's year-long, trying illness. In that year his business collapsed, their only child married and left home, and he finally died. She was left tired, alone, financially insecure, and with the habit of drinking to keep going. It took time, patience, and a good deal of support and encouragement on my part to help her regain health and energy, find a job, make new friends, and eventually become rested and secure enough to keep going on her own inner strengths.

The woman who has all her life depended for security on her youth and beauty sometimes turns to alcohol as she grows older and feels less attractive.

'A drink buoys me up,' insisted one such patient to me. 'I forget how I looked in the mirror. I feel as gay as a girl again on the dance floor.'

'What's your husband doing while you're being gay as a girl?' I asked.

'Oh, either looking patient and kind of long-suffering, or else ignoring me completely.' Trying hard to be clever to cover up the hurt feelings, I thought.

'Look,' I said, 'when you get to a certain age you're going to have lines in your face and neck. All women do. Your husband loves *you*, not your complexion. Stop trying to get more attention from him by behaving like a girl. Learn what it's like to be cherished because you're a *woman*.'

The challenge intrigued her. A few months later I saw her with her husband at a dinner-party. Instead of the 'cute little girl' creations she had affected, she wore a tastefully selected gown which was exactly right for her. Best of all, her animation was genuine, her face serene – and her husband was conspicuously attentive!

The problem of sleep has given birth to whole new industries, scientific experiments, millions of words on paper (to which I am about to add!), and many controversies. I tell my patients to pay plenty of attention to the amount of rest they require, but never to worry about how much sleep they get. For most people the problem arises from anxieties which are part of the age we live in, and the real solution is in learning to live with anxiety. A difficult task, all right, but the reward is a self-assurance we will never win by relying on drugs.

The fatigue that urges you to seek sleep is to be welcomed. It is the body's signal for help in keeping a balance of energy, the balance between wear and repair. People have trouble responding to the signal because they have difficulty with muscles that ache instead of letting go, and with nervous systems that remain over-active. Some sleeping pills or tranquillizers help relax muscles, some cut down alertness to stimuli in the environment.

Most people enjoy sleeping, though on the face of it it does seem to be a waste of time. The experts can't tell us exactly what happens during sleep. It seems to put things in a better perspective. Worries and fears never look as bad in the morning as they did the night before. This power of sleep to set our world in order seems to have more to do with the quality of sleep than its duration. Sometimes a five-minute nap completely changes our outlook; then again, a ten-hour sleep leaves us tired and drowsy.

Many people worry about their sleep, feel that they must get a certain number of hours in, or need a lot more than other people. It is not worth arguing about, because the amount of sleep we need depends partly on our habits. If you interrupt your regular life by going someplace else for a few days to visit, vacation, or do business, you find it difficult to stay awake past your usual bedtime for a few nights. This is true even for people who are poor sleepers.

It is wise to plan reasonable regularity of a time to go to bed and to get up. Strangely enough, the importance of this is seldom realized by people who claim difficulty in getting to sleep. Something else to remember is that if you are happy, you cannot possibly lose too much sleep. When our bodies really need sleep, unless there is some worry or frustration gnawing at us, it is almost impossible to resist the mechanism by which the body turns off our awareness and drops us into oblivion.

The depth of sleep varies with your frame of mind, even as the emotional state may determine the ease with which you drop off. If you don't go to sleep right away after you have had coffee at a party, it is likely the stimulation of the company rather than the caffeine that keeps you awake. In any case, it's not a bad thing to relax, rest, and review the evening you've had, especially if it's been a pleasant one, while you wait for your emotional tone to ease down so that sleep can fold you away.

Many young mothers become completely tired out because they have not slept soundly during the prolonged illness of a child, or simply because they feel the responsibility to make sure the child is well covered. Again, I believe this is failure to relax tension. Experiments have shown that broken sleep is often more refreshing than continuous sleep. It really isn't harmful to have your sleep interrupted several times a night by your child, as long as you have a sense of basic security — a feeling that your child is going to be all right, and that you have done your best.

The change of pace from a busy day at work or at home helps to relax people and get them ready for a refreshing sleep. A few minutes' relaxation before dinnertime is good for everybody, especially mother or whoever is going to get dinner. Evenings at home should be a happy family time. Children like to know their parents are around while they are studying, and most people who work need several evenings a week at home to decompress the head of steam they carry all day. Reading or working at hobbies helps replace life's inevitable frustrations with the happy satisfactions of small accomplishments. Sleep comes easily to those who have had a relaxing, interesting evening.

On the nights when we work late, attend meetings, or do something else which doesn't mean relaxation or recreation, sometimes interest or tension carries over and makes it harder to go to sleep. If it doesn't happen too frequently, this does no harm; most people can go on for several nights without their usual amount of sleep. In fact, it may even do good, if a person feels the time has been well spent and the accomplishments will contribute something good to her home, family or profession.

We must be matter-of-fact about this: in our age and our society, it takes time to relax. The change of pace, the change of interest, taking a warm bath, listening to a little favourite music, doing some little job with our hands – there are many techniques, and each of us must find the ones that will be satisfactory for us. But there is a way.

The human organism has ways of helping us to be alert, to relax, to sleep, and to withstand physical and emotional stress. We must work with nature's gifts, not against them, in order to be at our best. A short cut may promise much in the beginning but will fail us in the end.

12

Trapped by Her Own Adaptability

YOU CAN HAVE whatever you want from life. I believed this when I started off to university in 1920. I still believe it.

My mother gave me a good tip on how to start. 'Enter every open door,' she said. (When I asked her if she didn't think this might have some intriguing consequences, she didn't know what I meant.) It's been awfully good advice. Opportunity has seldom had to knock more than once for me. Along with the rest of the human race, I have had to learn, however, how to distinguish between a genuine opportunity and a red herring!

Now, nearly four decades later, I must add something to that neat sentence: You can have whatever you want — if you are willing to pay the price. The price is this: being a person all your life.

Nature sees to it that a woman plays many roles in the successive stages of her life. She's a flirt, a sweetheart, a wife, a mother, a lover. Some roles belong to a definite period of time. The time for flirting is when she is young and playing the field. As a girl grows up and moves into a real love relationship and closer to marriage, her role as a flirt becomes a minor one. Others roles call for peak performances interchangeably in the same period of time. At a certain stage of life a woman may be all wife one moment, all mother the next. The secret of her quick-change artistry is her wondrous adaptability.

Women have two main streams in life: the biological and the personal. Today the personal stream of life is being affected by many economic and social changes. Daily, women are confronted with new demands. They keep too busy meeting immediate demands to do the assessing and priority setting that are necessary for successful long-range adaptation. This generation of women is having to feel its way through today's changes. The generation that is just embarking on life will be able to predict more of what may happen to them and plan for it.

Take the question of women working. Women have always worked, and *hard*, but always as a contribution to an institution of which they were a part – the family. Now they work outside the home, for money and for someone else. Although the number of women in the labour market has increased astonishingly and definite patterns of women's employment are emerging, the fact that this is part of our way of life and will continue to be has not yet fully penetrated into the minds of women.

College girls take their education somewhat for granted and look forward principally to marrying and raising a family. They know what the statistics say about working women, but each thinks they refer to other college girls and not herself. The fact is that most women will work until they marry, probably afterward until they begin to have a family, and again after their children are grown. Today's college girl must get the best education she possibly can, not only to enhance her ability to make a happy marriage and raise a family intelligently, but also because the chances are that she will work. Her future happiness and capacity for personal achievement are at stake.

My phrase of diagnosis for the woman who is pulled apart by all the things that are demanded of her is that she's trapped by her own adaptability. Down through the centuries woman has had to be adaptable. Her adaptability comes naturally from her female nature. (One could wish that sometimes, particularly in the area of love-making, she would just *be* natural and not talk about it so much!)

It is not just that women adapt themselves to the female nature and the requirements of life with or without a family. A woman can – must – also adapt herself to her environment; when it changes, she must change.

One theme song that has been dinned monotonously into our ears for far too long is that one that begins 'the changing role of modern women'. There is no doubt about it that a woman's role has changed. But too many speeches and articles seem to imply that women must wait until the dust settles or their role stops evolving, before they can hope to grapple with the situation.

I believe women should, and can, deal adequately and happily with all the changes in their world and their family relationships right now, today.

It is astonishing to me that women are so slow to grasp this challenge.

I have a tremendous admiration for them. You just need to see a mother defending her child to know they are not only brave, but can have steel in their souls. You just need to look at the history of certain social changes such as laws against child labour or laws for woman suffrage to know they can also have a crusade in their hearts.

But along with the steel in her soul and the crusading heart, a woman has the capacity for great gentleness and complete capitulation of her body.

Here you have a living, breathing human creature with all these natural gifts. Why is it she has not learned to use them to bring herself a truly happy life? Why has she not sorted out the things in our changing life that are affecting her and decided what she will do about them?

A woman's amazing ability to adapt gives her a real versatility. She can manage her life in several different ways – if she knows what she's doing and can catch on to the object of the game! It's easy for her to get confused, because her life is never the same from one year to another.

When her children are small, a mother never has them off her mind a minute. She must try to arrange her life so that she does not have too many other stresses, especially during the day when the children are awake and requiring constant attention. She should have help with the housework if it is at all possible, and I hope she is lucky

enough to have one or two people – family or neighbours – with whom she can leave the children for an
afternoon or evening and feel reasonably comfortable
about it.

The children start to school and the mother enters
what one of my patients called 'the best years of your
life'. She has the day to herself, comparatively speaking.
She can go to morning coffee parties and Home and
School of Parent-Teacher Association meetings. She
gets more rest, has more fun. But from now on until the
children are grown up, she must be ready to be on the
job from the time school is out until bedtime.

With the children in the teen-age years, she has a
different set of stresses. They are growing up. They
have many decisions to make – about school, about
dating, about life and how to live it. She must be ready
to help, wise about not expecting too much of them, yet
able to hold herself together while they inch up to the
independence they will need.

When the children have left home to marry or work,
again she must examine her whole life situation and decide how she will spend her time and concentrate her interests. The stresses will have diminished and she will
have to be her own self-starter. One of my patients re-
decorated her home from top to bottom as a beginning
for this new phase of her life. Another took a course in
anthropology, a subject which had always interested
her, and joined a summer crew of amateurs digging for
Indian relics.

This is why I say women in different circumstances

should never compare themselves with each other; their problems are different.

The crux of the trouble is not that woman is too adaptable or too versatile. It is that she allows herself to be trapped by her adaptability rather than remaining mistress of it. She gets mixed up in her roles. Sometimes she puts all her emphasis on being a mother, and wraps herself around her children. Or she may put all her emphasis on being a wife and wrap herself around her husband. Again, she may drift into being all employee, and let her job become the touchstone of her life.

My plea is for women to be women, and for women always to be themselves.

From the time a woman is born until she dies she is not only a woman but also a person. All persons have basic human needs. The basic need for every woman is to have a central core inside herself, a centre and a strength that is entirely her own.

Without this she's going to be whatever turns up – what the economy asks, or what the men think beautiful, or what the children want to make them happy. My idea of negative thinking (or, perhaps, no thinking at all) is to allow oneself to be propelled by the demands from the environment. This is how people get into a mad race where they have the eerie feeling they're running pell-mell just to stay in place.

As a woman, you can run the gamut of all the roles you must play in life, but you always come back to this: you can have what you want if you are willing to pay the price of being a person all your life. A woman should never make the error of considering herself a wife, or a mother, or a widow, or a divorcee. She is a person above all – a whole person with all the wealth of attributes which being a woman embodies.

In this high-powered, tense, specialized civilization, women's responsibilities are difficult and complicated. They must be the same constant, unwearying bulwark of the home. At the same time they must begin to learn to move out into the community and the world.

The truth is that the world needs women to be persons rather than females playing various roles upon demand. We are in a transitional period today, a great social upheaval. Aside from what's happening in other parts of the world, here on our own continent there are rapid changes calling for adjustments women must learn to make intelligently. In the Eastern countries women are waking up to themselves. Women in the Western countries forged ahead for a while; now they seem to have reached a plateau.

There never was a better time to be a woman.

I believe – and this is the real reason I want women to lick the fatigue problem – that women can and will find their way through this changing world, that they will reach the stature and attainments for which they were created, and that this will be a sensitive, knowledgeable, and stabilizing force in this unhappy, dislocated world.

A woman may say, 'But I don't want struggle and achievement. I just want to be happy.' She doesn't realize that happiness is a by-product of maturity. Maturity is the ability to meet whatever life offers with intelligence and faith, and that doesn't mean just the courage to cope with bad breaks, but the grace and dignity to take the lucky breaks too.

Real maturity lies in achieving a basis of survival. I am not speaking of physical survival. I mean the survival of self, the person. Stripped of all the accompaniments of adulthood which we so often mistake for maturity – possessions, status, acquaintances, responsibilities – we must feel that there is a strong central core of self remaining.

A psychologist could easily supply a fine, precise definition of maturity. But I think what I mean is expressed best in my favourite *Good Friday* poem by John Masefield:

I had a valley farm above a brook,
My sheep bells there were sweet,
And in the summer heat
My mill wheels turned, yet all these things they took;
Ah, and I gave them, all things I forsook
But that green blade of wheat.
My own soul's courage, that they did not take.

13

'Love God and Do as You Please'

I STAND AT the surgeons' room on the top floor of our hospital looking out across the city as the sun rises. There's a murmur of voices in the background, as the doctors and anaesthetists sit around talking of this case or that one. I stand apart. The night has been long, as I have watched over my patient going through her labour. Now it is gradually becoming clear that nature is not going to be able to work out this miracle of birth. This is the moment for decision; something must be done.

As I watch the sun rise, in an instant of agonized projection of spirit I feel the great gap close, the gap between the everyday reality of the hospital ward and the great infinity, the power of God. Even as I stand there, inarticulate but full of faith, the answer comes back: 'Be still, keep quiet, just do your best. I am God.'

Anxiety and indecision pass away. I go in to my patient and say, 'This is the time. Now we are going to have the baby.' I go downstairs to the father, who is waiting anxiously, and say, 'Hang on tight. This is the moment we have been waiting for.' I go back to my patient. There is a special feeling about this moment. There seems to be a communication deeper than words. Patient and doctor are at one with the life and force of creation. There is faith that this will go well, but there is no guarantee that the deep-felt hope will be fulfilled.

These moments of great spiritual need, response, and awareness of resource are not everyday occurrences but when they do come, they are so vivid, so exciting, so full of peace, that their reality and the memory of them go on and on and on. Every obstetrician has known these moments of grave danger and great exhilaration.

Every surgeon knows the wonder of coming into the operating-room before the patient is put to sleep. Each in his own particular fashion gives a greeting to communicate to the patient the sense of faithfulness and the presence of a caring heart as well as an expert hand. No one is ever too busy, too preoccupied, or too much in a hurry to give that extra faith to patients in their hour of need.

A great many of my patients that I operate on are older women. When they come to the operating-room their false teeth have been removed, so that they lie with hand over mouth, feeling very self-conscious, retreating from being recognized. Yet inevitably these patients say afterwards, 'Oh, Doctor, I was so glad to hear your voice.'

This kind of complete communication between patient and doctor can be almost a total revelation of one to another. It does not depend on the length of time they have known each other. It depends on the need of the moment and on the faith of both – the faith of the patient in her doctor, the doctor's faith that he will do his best. We all understand these moments. Some of them are unforgettable. Both the great moments of desperate need and the more everyday moments of communication in the operating-room or the delivery-room are the highlights of a doctor's life.

If anyone asked me what part of my practice of medicine over the last thirty years had been the most rewarding to *me*, I would have to say they were those hours I had spent in the delivery-room. If anyone asked what part of my work had been most rewarding to my *patients*, I would have to say it was the long, hard, slugging office hours I have put in over the years.

Each patient comes to the office with new problems and a new difficulty. Each is asking for your complete attention and all you have to give in skill, competence, and experience. The treatment detailed for the patient when the examination is over is not the most important part of the office visit, though of course it is important that it be accurate, definite, and in accordance with the best known therapy of the day. But this is only the beginning. The most important thing is that this person who has come for help shall have the faith to carry out what is written down on those little pieces of paper. She has to be helped to have that faith. Sometimes she is preoccupied and already really has her mind on the next thing she has to do – stop at the grocery store, pick up the children at school, get her husband's suit at the drycleaner's, or hurry back to her office. Then you have to sit her down, look her in the eye, and say, in some way or other, 'Relax and quiet down. Listen to me. This is what you must do.'

Sometimes the doctor is preoccupied, busy, pressed for time. Then he may fail to communicate the spirit of faith to the patient and nothing much will happen. Even when the preoccupation is of a serious nature and the busy-ness and hurry have life-and-death overtones, the doctor must try to remember that this moment of need for faith and communication is as important as the moment of entering the operating-room. Because I believe this so deeply, I keep trying, and when the preoccupation has been too great and I have short-cut the time a little, I have an inward feeling of sorrow that my patient and I have missed this moment.

The success or failure in treatment, like the success or failure of life, depends on a person's faith and trust in the purpose of his or her own life.

'Mother, why is it that you're so nervous when you talk to me about sex or religion?' asked the fourteen-year-old daughter of one of my patients.

'Why, I'm not nervous when I talk to you,' replied her mother, somewhat taken aback by this rather acute question.

'Oh, yes you are.'

'How do you know?'

'Because when you talk about those things your voice rises half a key,' said the youngster calmly.

Recounting the incident to me, the mother said, 'She's right, of course. I don't know what I'm going to do about it. I don't know why it's so hard.'

'I know why,' I told her. 'When you're talking about sex or religion you're talking about the great creative powers of life. It's easy for such power to overwhelm you, get away from your control, so you hate to start it. Try talking about it simply, then you won't get nervous.'

'But how can you be simple about these things?' she asked wonderingly.

A small incident, but it set me to meditating.

Today most families spend their lives on a humdrum, repetitive merry-go-round full of frustrations, just like the office hours of a doctor. Though there may be no great highlights of tragedy, excitement, or danger, their lives are full of uneasiness, and they are fearful of the future. I think back to life in my family when I was growing up. We always had a great sense of adventure, a feeling that there was a great destiny for each of us. My mother had the most amazing capacity for making us feel we had been called to some great endeavour.

Life now seems to have become so complex, so full of sound and electronics, that most women try to avoid the entanglements that go along with the great endeavours of this age. Mothers bring up their children in health and wealth as best they can. They are always anxious to do as well as they should, and as well as their neighbours. They try their best to follow the rules and examples laid down by experts in magazine articles and books. No generation of women ever have tried harder. And no generation of women have been so pulled apart by their efforts. It is as though the problems of the world have become so great, so complicated, that women have given up trying to understand enough so they can help their

children deal with pressures of the world that are beyond
the home. So they do their best with ideas which happen
to be going the rounds on the block or in their town or
suburban village. It may bother them at times that they
do not understand the theory of Einstein or the political
importance of the Middle East, but it is easy to decide
that these things are beyond the scope of one's life.

At this moment in our history I believe we would do
well to listen across the centuries to the voice of St
Augustine. 'Love God and do as you please' is a kind of
free translation of a remark he made in Latin in his writ-
ings about the Gospel of St John. I believe this sentence
sums it up. It is the answer, the way a modern woman
can cope with her difficult, complex, theory-ridden environment, the way a mother can do her best for her
children.

As soon as you love God, you realize at once that
this is God's world and you don't need to be afraid;
you do your best.

When you love God and your spirit goes swinging
out to close that gap between those things you can see
and the wonder of the Spirit that you can feel, you know
you do not have to depend entirely on your own resources.

If you love God, then you must come apart from life
and look at it, look at your own life to see just where it is
going. Then you can see where the adventure is, where
the sense of destiny is. You will know that we are called
into this life not for what we can get, but that we are
created to love, to give. There is rest and refreshment

for the person who takes some time each day to look at the value of life, to feel again the joy that comes from the inner knowledge that she is loved by God.

During the last decades, through the growth of psychiatry and its knowledge of the disturbed personality, we have learned about the necessity for being rid of that great bundle of guilt that most of us carry. It has been a wonderful relief for mankind to have learned so much about the necessity of finding its way through this and, as it were, coming through to a sense that its sins are forgiven.

But if we stop here, we have missed another part of life. It is important that we shall not only have a sense that our sins are forgiven and that we are rid of our guilt feelings, but that we also have a sense of the overwhelming joy coming from the fact that we belong in a world where God is our Father, where we are loved.

Somehow or other in our preoccupations with the small things of life, many of us have not grasped the glorious sense of adventuring in faith, nor come to the knowledge that there is this great power of love which catches us up. For those who have, the drive of competition and the urgent need to go one step better than their neighbours has given way before the knowledge that the greatest value we have in life is the fact that we are children of God. Once we find that this is so for us, then all the false values and the greed for material security are gone, and we walk with grace and with a sense of the dignity of life.

Those who love God keep his commandments.

That's why St Augustine could say, 'Love God and do as you please.' Because then it becomes your pleasure to love your neighbour and to think first of the other person. It becomes your great delight to be part of the power of loving in the world.

It means that a mother will not be preoccupied with busy-ness, but will be sensitive and alert to the needs and problems of her children and her husband. She will become a channel for the spirit of love which inevitably brings serenity and peace to those who are in need.

It means that every worker, whether she is on the maintenance staff or the head of the company, is of equal value in life, simply because of her joy that she can contribute to the well-being of those with whom she works. We all have different functions at different levels of society; the value of what we are ourselves can only be judged by what we can contribute through love to the comfort and happiness of those with whom we associate.

It means that we will be able to give ourselves in real commitment to ideas and undertakings that are bigger than ourselves and our own small concerns. Losing our small selves in big causes and concerns for which we work with others, we truly find ourselves.

Every person must have a home, a room of his own, a resting place where life is restored. I think you can tell when you enter a house whether or not it is really a home, a place where family members gain strength and peace for the journey of life. The purpose of parents is not to make the way easy for their children; it is to make a home where the children gain knowledge and security, where they may hear the call to the adventure of living. In such a home a child becomes strong, so that when he meets the inevitably difficult times in life, he will be able to have a small victory within himself, regardless of how the difficulty turns out.

If we want to master the fearful and frustrating drive of our modern life and the enormous weariness which comes in its wake, we must get straight what life is about. We must find the dynamic force of life and become a part of it.

Like my patient, we have trouble talking about loving God. It's too hot to handle. It has so much dynamic power in it that we pull away from it. Yet this is where our hope lies; this is where fear ends, where faith and joy begin; this is where we find strength for striving, courage for acceptance of the inevitable. This is where we find a constant joy, a constant adventure, a constant peace.

Love God and do as you please. If you do, fatigue vanishes.

INDEX

Index

Abortion, 44
Achievement, 12, 83, 150; need for, 130; sense of, 124, 125
Adaptability: to environment, 150, of women, 148–55; trap for women, 153
Adaptation, 34
Adjustment, happiness and, 34
Adolescence, 12, 13, 18, 20, 22, 37, 49, 50, 60; going steady, 69–70, 78–79; metabolism and, 50–51. See also Teenagers
Adrenal gland, 19
Advertising, effect on modern life, 125
Affection, 82; need for, 127, 130
Africa, 115
Ageing, 80–84; rigidity of, 82
Alcohol, 138–43; examples, 141–4; fatigue and, 139; nervous system, 140; unhappiness and, 139
Alcoholics, 86, 139–40
Anxiety, living with, 144
Apathy, 13
Arguments, 20
Arthritic tendency, overweight and, 89

Arthritis, 22
Assault, 17

Backaches, 11, 18, 23; causes of, 99–100, 101
Banting, Dr, 27
Behaviour, basis of, 23
Benzedrine, 134
Best, Dr, 27
Birth, 18
Blood vessels, fatigue and, 36
Body temperature, raising, 24
Boredom: alcohol and, 139; in love-making, 110

Cause and effect, law of, 17
Chain smoking, 139
Chest, fatigue and, 36
Childbearing, 50
Childbirth, 17; fatigue after, 92, 93
Childhood, 18
Childlessness, 46
Children: desire for, 116–17; needs of, 94
China, 115
Communication, doctor-patient, 157–8
Companionship, 126
Compassion, 113–14

Conception, time element for, 43

Cortisone, 22–23

Coward, Noel, 84

Creation, 157

Death, 18; fear of, 58

Delivery, 58

Development, law of, 18

Diabetics, 86

Diet: fad, 87; fatigue and, 87

Dieting, 88

'Doctor-shopping,' 42

Drinking, See Alcohol

Drive, 13; of modern civilization, 119–20, 121

Drugs, 136

Education, women and, 72–73, 102, 115–16, 149–50

Emotional balance, menopause and, 61

Emotions, effect on metabolic cycle, 31

Endocrine system, 19

Energy: demand-production relationship, 25; dynamism of, 16–17; evaluation of, 33; individual patterns of, 28–29; menopause and, 63, 65; metabolic pattern and, 26; metabolism and, 19; pituitary gland and, 21; understanding limit of, 25

Environment, adaptability to, 150, 154

Excesses: dangers of, 139–40; making virtues of, 139

Exercise, 89–90

Exhaustion, 28, 29, 30, 37; causes of, 32

Faith, 83, 157, 162

Family life, 91–103; happiness factors, 101–3; modern, 115–33. See also Modern life

Family patterns, contemporary, 115 ff.

Family relations, mother's fatigue and, 91 ff.

Fatherhood, fatigue in, 59

Fatigue: after accomplishment, 32; adolescence and, 12, apathy and, 13; in contemporary culture, 134; control of, 97; 'doctor-shopping,' 42; eating and, 90; effect on women, 12; enjoyment of, 32; faces of, 36–47; factors, 13; faith and, 164; female biology and, 37, 50; female vulnerability to, 12; from fighting age, 80; frustration and, 25; inevitability of, 12; menopause and, 12, 59–66; example, 30–31; natural, 13; pregnancy and, 12, 53–59; prevention, 32; problem, 15; reasons for, 12–13; social changes and, 12; -stress relationship, 28; time element, importance of, 29; troublesome kind, 32; women's greatest enemy, 11. See also Energy

Fatigue patterns, 25, 27

Fear: of love, 76; stress of, 58

Female biology, and fatigue, 50

Fertility, 46
Flushing, 62
Food faddists, 87
Food requirements, 87
Fortitude, in women, 48–49
Frailty, in women, 48–66
Friendship, 71; platonic, 130
Frustration, 13, 45, 46; fatigue and, 25

General adaptation syndrome, 28
Glandular change, 35
Glandular system, 19, 20; changes in (female), 22
God, love of, 161–4
Going steady, 69–70, 79
Greece, 38
Guilt, 44, 47, 162

Happiness: adjustment and, 33; maturity and, 155
Headaches, 11, 18, 38
Haemorrhages, 62
Heredity, 18; energy and, 26; metabolic pattern, 21, 26
High-metabolism, example, 24
Hippocrates, 16
Honeymoons, 106
Hormone activity, 22
Hormones, 19, 20

India, 115
Infection, 11, 18, 23
Infertility, 43–47
Insulin, 27
Insult, 17
Irregular bleeding, 62

Joints: fatigue and, 36; overweight and, 88

Kinsey, Dr Alfred, 109

Labour, 56, 58
Lassitude, 16, 28
Life: rhythm of, 67–84; struggle in, 68
Life cycle, 18, 49–50; energy and, 66
Life force, 45
Liquor, 134. See also Alcohol
Loneliness, 13, 126–30; fatigue and, 126, 127, 138
Love, 31, 40, 46, 75; boredom and, 110; and family life, 103; fatigue and, 104–14; of God, 161–4; -passion, confusion of, 130–32; -passion, differences between, 132–3; power of, 114; separation and, 110. See also Sex relations
Love-making, 54; boredom in, 110; distractions in, 108; love in, 133; wife's interest in, 106–8; women and, 150
Low-metabolism, example, 23–24

Malnutrition, 86–87
Marriage, 75, 76–80; compassion in, 113–14; consummation of, 44; early, 116; happiness factors, 102–3; weaknesses of, 110–12
Masefield, John, 155
Materialistic values, example, 120–23

Maternity leaves, 56

Maturity, 18, 83; happiness and, 154–5

Menopause, 12, 18, 20, 22, 38, 49, 50; emotional balance, 61; energy and, 63, 65; fluctuations of, 61; uncertainty of, 41; fatigue in, 59–66; example, 30–31; menstruation and, 62; metabolism and, 50; pregnancy and, 46; sex relations and, 109; sex life in, 109; sympathy and, 65; time of, 60; transition stage, 83; understanding of, 62–64

Menstrual cycle, 12, 50

Menstrual disturbances, example, 38–39, 128

Menstruation, 18, 23, 112; disorders, 36; disturbances, fatigue and, 38; menopause and, 62; pain and, 38

Metabolic cycles: changes in, 31; examples, 23–25

Metabolic pattern, 19, 20; differences of, 20; heredity and, 21, 26

Metabolism, 19, 24; abrupt changes and, 31; females, cycles in, 50; glandular changes and, 50; pregnancy and, 53; raising, 31

Miscarriage, 55, 56

Modern life: complexity of, 160 pitfalls of, 118 ff.

Morrisburg, Ontario, 98

Mother: fatigue in, 91 ff.; role in family life, 103

Motherhood, 37, 53; age for, 101–2; fatigue in, 59; outside interests, necessity of, 98 ff.

National Manpower Council, 117

Natural fatigue, 13

Nature: fatigue of fighting, 84; power of, 16, 67; timing of, 67; always the winner, 84

Nauseousness, 38

Neededness, 83

Nervousness, 136–7

Nervous system, 19, 20; alcohol and, 139; changes in (female), 22; pattern of, 22; rhythm of, 22

Neuroglandular activity: intensity of, 20; timing of, 20

Neuroglandular system, 19

Nutrition, 85–86; fatigue and, 86

Obstetrics, 34

Old age, 18

Old age pension, 100

Overeating: continuous, 88; fatigue and, 88

Overweight: danger of, 90; exercise and, 89–90; fatigue and, 88

Pace, changing of, 97, 123; fatigue and, 32

Pain, 58

Parenthood, time for, 101

Parents, purpose of, 163

Passion: -love, confusion of, 130–2; -love, differences between, 132–3

Pituitary gland, 19, 21
Platonic friendship, 130
Pregnancy, 12, 22, 37, 43, 53–59; arthritis and, 22; fear in, 58; menopause and, 46; metabolism and, 50, 53; miscarriages, percentage of, 56; 'rabbit test,' 60
Psychiatry, 162
Puberty, 18

Recreation, 97
Relaxation, 147; techniques for, 147
Responsibility, towards old folk, 100–1
Rest, importance of, 95 ff.; timing, importance of, 97
Rheumatic tendency, overweight and, 89
Rhythm, of life, 67–84

St Augustine, 161, 163
Self-assessment, necessity of, for women, 14
Selye, Dr Hans, 27–28
Separation, 110
Sex, 75–76; fear of, 76
Sex glands, 19, 50
Sex life, energy factor, 105
Sex relations: boredom, 110; after childbirth, 109; male interest decline, 109; menopause and, 109; withholding, 110
Shakespeare, William, 48
Shame, infertility and, 44
Short cuts: artificiality of, 137 fallacy of, 134–47

Skin rash, 36
Sleep, 144–7; power of, 145; quality factor, 145; tension and, 147
Sleeping pills, 134, 144
Social changes, fatigue and, 12
Status, need for, 130
Stimulants, 138
Stress, 27; defined, 28; -fatigue relationship, 28; history, 29; juggling, 97; laws of, 52
Stress factors, 28, 33
Stressful activities, effect on metabolic cycle, 31
Stressors, 28
Sympathy, 65

Teen-agers, 51–53; basic needs of, 71–72; emotional maturity, 69; learning time, 69; roots, importance of, 73
Tension, 34–35, 136; pain and, example, 38–39; sleep and, 147
Thyroid gland, 19
Time element, importance in fatigue, 29
Time-energy, budget, 95
Timing, 67; adult responsibility, 74–75; importance of, in fatigue, 97
Tiredness, 41
Tranquillizers, 138, 144

University of Toronto, 27
Unhappiness, alcohol and, 140
Unmarried women, 128–30; love and, 108

Vitality, fallacy of short cuts for, 134–47

Women: adaptability of, 148–55; composite role of, 153–4; education for, 72–73, 102, 115–16, 149–50; employment of, 117; individuality of problems, 153; important needs of, 83; post-menopause, 50; reasons for wanting children, 117; roles of, 12, 49–50, 148–9; self-understanding, lack of, 33; unmarried, 128–9; vulnerability to fatigue, 12; working, 149; percentage, 117; working wives, 78

Work, stimulus of, 34

Working mother, 94–99, 96; rest and, 96–97

Working women, self-assessment, 123

World War II, 38

Youth, flexibility of, 82

Health and Family Affairs

Dr. David Kellett Carding
THE HOME MEDICAL GUIDE   30p
Dr. A. Ward Gardner & Dr. Peter J.
Roylance
NEW SAFETY AND FIRST-AID   30p
NEW ESSENTIAL FIRST-AID   30p
Dr. Haim G. Ginott
BETWEEN PARENT AND CHILD   25p
Rose Hacker
THE OPPOSITE SEX   25p
D. C. Jarvis, M.D.
FOLK MEDICINE   25p
Dr. Winifred de Kok
YOUR BABY AND YOU (illus.)   30p
Amram Scheinfeld
THE BASIC FACTS OF HUMAN
HEREDITY   30p
Edited by Dr. Linton Snaith &
Dr. Alan Coxon
DICK READ'S CHILDBIRTH
WITHOUT FEAR (illus.)   37½p
Irwin Maxwell Stillman, M.D., &
Samm Sinclair Baker
THE DOCTOR'S QUICK WEIGHT
LOSS DIET   25p

Philosophy and Psychology

Havelock Ellis
PSYCHOLOGY OF SEX   25p
John Fowles
THE ARISTOS   30p
Arthur Koestler
THE ACT OF CREATION   75p
THE GHOST IN THE MACHINE   75p
Geoffrey Parrinder
THE WORLD'S LIVING
RELIGIONS   25p
William Sargant
BATTLE FOR THE MIND   30p
THE UNQUIET MIND   45p
Robert H. Thouless
STRAIGHT AND CROOKED
THINKING   25p
Colin Wilson
THE OUTSIDER   35p

Pan Reference

EVERYMAN'S ROGET'S
THESAURUS   65p
Edited by D. C. Browning
A DICTIONARY OF FAMOUS
QUOTATIONS   37½p
Compiled by Robin Hyman
ENGLISH PROVERBS EXPLAINED   25p
Ronald Ridout & Clifford Witting
BETTER ENGLISH   25p
G. H. Vallins
THE BEST ENGLISH   30p
G. H. Vallins
CASSELL'S COMPACT ENGLISH
DICTIONARY   60p
CASSELL'S COMPACT
FRENCH-ENGLISH
ENGLISH-FRENCH DICTIONARY   60p
CASSELL'S COMPACT
GERMAN-ENGLISH
ENGLISH-GERMAN DICTIONARY   50p
CAREERS FOR BOYS   40p
Gavin Brown
CAREERS FOR GIRLS   40p
Gavin Brown
GUIDE TO INSURANCE   30p
W. A. Dinsdale
THE PAN BOOK OF DOGS (illus.)   30p
Catherine Fisher
HOW TO STUDY   30p
Harry Madox
GUIDE TO LETTER WRITING   30p
K. Graham Thomson
HOW TO BE AN EFFECTIVE
SECRETARY   30p
Lance Secretan

Sports and Pastimes

100 YEARS OF THE F.A. CUP:
The Official Centenary History (illus.)
Tony Pawson   95p
THE PAN BOOK OF CHESS
Gerald Abrahams   30p
NEEDLEWORK AND EMBROIDERY
(illus.) Winifred Butler   25p
THE COMPLETE PATIENCE BOOK
Basil Dalton   30p
THE PAN BOOK OF WINE MAKING
(illus.) B. C. A. Turner   25p
THE PAN BOOK OF CARD GAMES
Hubert Phillips   30p
HOW TO DRAW (illus.)
Adrian Hill   30p
THE BEST PARTY GAMES
Joseph Edmundson   25p
STAMPS FOR INVESTMENT (illus.)
Kenneth Lake   30p
HOW TO PLAY A GOOD GAME OF
BRIDGE
Terence Reese & Albert Dormer   30p